Gastric Band Hypnosis for Rapid Weight Loss

2 Books in 1:

*Lose Weight Fast and Burn Fat with Intuitive Eating &
Stop Sugar Cravings. Mindful Eating & Crave Less Food
Effortlessly in a Few Steps.*

Gastric Band Hypnosis for Rapid Weight Loss

This Book Includes

Book 1:
Rapid Weight Loss Hypnosis
Lose Weight with a Natural and Rapid Weight Loss Journey. Learn Powerful Hypnosis, Meditations, Motivation, Self Esteem, Mindful Eating and Mini Habits.

Book 2:
Extreme-Rapid Weight Loss Hypnosis
Eat Healthy with Rapid Weight Loss Hypnosis and Stop Food Addiction with, Meditation, Self Esteem, Powerful Habits, Mindful Eating and Self-Hypnosis.

Text Copyright ©

Legal & Disclaimer

Rapid Weight Loss Hypnosis

Lose Weight with a Natural and Rapid Weight Loss Journey. Learn Powerful Hypnosis, Meditations, Motivation, Self Esteem, Mindful Eating and Mini Habits.

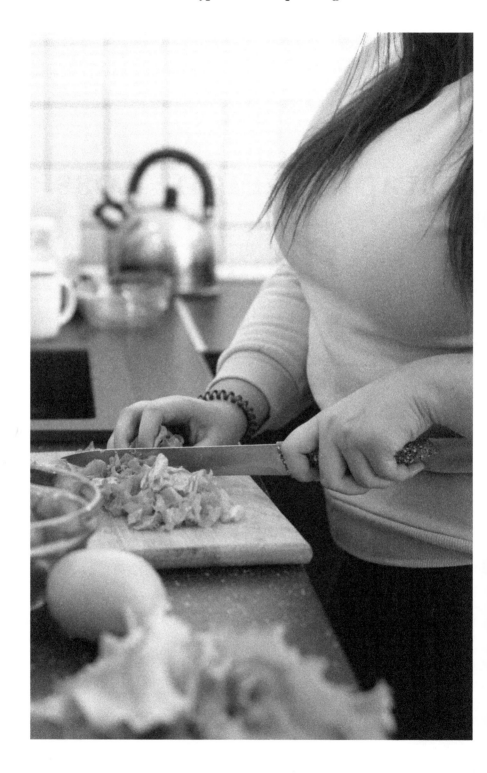

Table of Contents

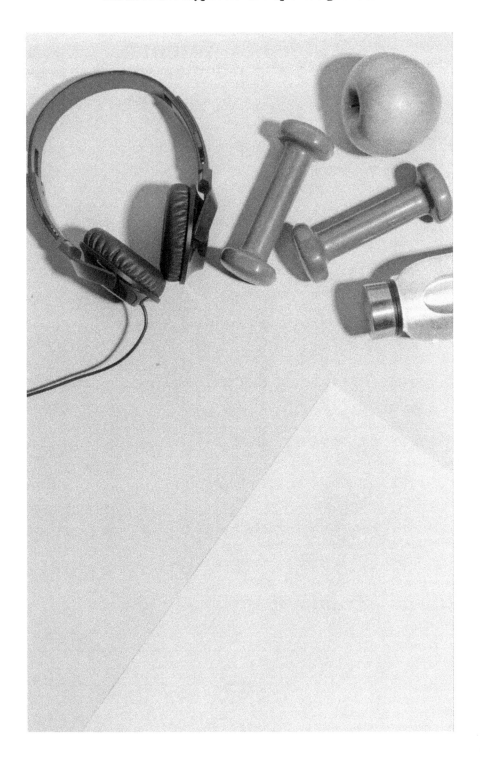

INTRODUCTION

What you will find in this book

D o you struggle to lose weight? Have you always visualized yourself as thin, attractive, and free from any health conditions brought on by excess weight? Do you desire to get certain things in your life, only to feel held back by the body that you have?

Throughout this book, we have provided you with four different mindset exercises in order to help you lose weight. These are hypnosis, meditations, and affirmations that will make it easier for you to rewire your brain so that you're focused on achieving your goals and getting the things that you want from this life.

Make sure that you do not do any of these meditations while you're driving or operating a motor vehicle. The best place possible for these meditations is in your home, in a place where you are completely relaxed and at ease. You do not want to put yourself in a risky situation by doing this meditation somewhere that you can't fall asleep. After you know how you react to these meditations, you might be able to do them in public, such as riding a train or an airplane for long periods of travel.

However, ensure that you understand how you might react, especially to hypnosis. Make sure that, as you're reading or listening to these meditations, you are focused on your breath, and keep an open mind. Letting your thoughts flow free can be the key to ensuring that you get the healthy body that you deserve.

Why you should read this book

If you are confused about the numerous deceptive weight loss measures in the world, then this book is the first step to take towards taking action about it. The first step is also always the easiest, which is you should take the information that you will find in the chapters dear to your heart as they include concepts that you can be put into action immediately. If you file them away until when you need them, then when the time comes actually to use them, you will be glad you did use them.

To that end, the following chapters in this book will discuss the hypnotic gastric band and put a special focus on using meditation and hypnosis to lose weight and start healthy eating. This means that you may want to consider making some changes to your subconscious mind about the perceptions that you have about your weight. Understanding the relevance of powerful affirmation and visualization, you will learn what it takes to get the body changes that you desire to make.

This means that you have to remain informed on why the hypnotic gastric band is the perfect solution to help you lose weight.

What is guided hypnosis

Hypnosis has always been surrounded by misconceptions and myths. In spite of being used clinically and all the research that has been done, some continue to be scared by the assumption that hypnosis is mystical. Many people think that hypnosis is a modern day innovation that spread through communities that believed in the metaphysical during the 70s and 80s. Since the mid-1800s, hypnosis was used in the United States. It has advanced with the help of psychologists such as Alfred Binet, Pierre Janet, and Sigmund Freud, and others. Hypnosis can be found in ancient times and has been investigated by modern researchers, physicians, and psychologists.

Hypnosis's origins can't be separated from psychology and western medicine. Most ancient cultures from Roman, Greek, Egyptian, Indian, Chinese, Persian, and Sumerian used hypnosis. In Greece and Egypt, people who were sick would go the places that healed. These were known as dream temples or sleep temples where people could be cured with hypnosis. The Sanskrit book called "The Law of Manu" described levels of hypnosis such as sleep-walking, dream sleep, and ecstasy sleep in ancient India.

The earliest evidence of hypnosis was found in the Egyptian Ebers Papyrus that dated back to 1550 BC. Priest/physicians repeated suggestions while treating patients. They would have the patient gaze at metal discs and enter a trance. This is now called eye fixation.

During the Middle Ages, princes and kings thought they could heal with the Royal Touch. These healings can be attributed to divine powers. Before people began to understand hypnosis, the terms mesmerism or magnetism would be used to describe this type of healing.

Paracelsus, the Swiss physician, began using magnets to heal. He didn't use a holy relic or divine touch. This type of healing was still being used in the 1700s. A Jesuit priest, Maximillian Hell was famous for healing using magnetic steel plates. Franz Mesmer, an Austrian physician, discovered he could send people into a trance without the use of magnets. He figured out the healing force came from inside himself or an invisible fluid that took up space. He thought that "animal magnetism" could be transferred from patient to healer by a mysterious etheric fluid. This theory is so wrong. It was based on ideas that were current during the time specifically Isaac Newton's theory of gravity.

Mesmer developed a method for hypnosis that was passed on to his followers. Mesmer would perform inductions by linking his patients together by a rope that the animal magnetism could pass over. He would also wear a cloak and play music on a glass harmonica while all this was happening. The image that a hypnotist was a mystical figure goes back to this.

These practices led to his downfall and for a time hypnotism was considered dangerous for anyone to have as a career. The fact remains that hypnosis works. The 19ᵗʰ century was full of people who were looking to understand and apply it.

Marquis de Puysegur, a student of Mesmer, was a successful magnetist who first used hypnosis called somnambulism or sleepwalking. Puysegur's followers called themselves experimentalists. Their work recognized that cures didn't come from magnets but from an invisible source.

Abbe Faria, an Indo-Portuguese priest, did hypnosis research in India during 1813. He went to Paris and studied hypnosis with Puysegur. He thought that hypnosis or magnetism wasn't what healed but the power that was generated from inside the mind.

His approach was what helped open the psychotherapy hypnosis centered school called Nancy School. The Nancy School said that hypnosis was a phenomenon brought on by the power of suggestion and not from magnetism. This school was founded by a French country doctor, Ambroise-Auguste Liebeault. He was called the father of modern hypnotherapy. He thought hypnosis was psychological and had nothing to do with magnetism. He studied the similar qualities of trance and sleep and noticed that hypnosis was a state that could be brought on by suggestion.

His book **Sleep and Its Analogous States** was printed in 1866. The stories and writings about his cures attracted Hippolyte Bernheim to visit him. Bernheim was a famous neurologist who was skeptical of

Liebeault, but once he observed Liebault, he was so intrigued that he gave up internal medicine and became a hypnotherapist. Bernhcim brought Liebeault's ideas to the medical world with **Suggestive Therapeutics** that showed hypnosis as a science. Bernheim and Liebeault were the innovators of psychotherapy. Even today, hypnosis is still viewed as a phenomenon.

The pioneers of psychology studied hypnosis in Paris and Nancy Schools. Pierre Janey developed theories of traumatic memory, dissociation, and unconscious processes studied hypnosis with Bernheim in Charcot in Paris and Nancy. Sigmund Freud studied hypnosis with Charcot and observed both Liebeault and Bernheim. Freud started practicing hypnosis in 1887. Hypnosis was critical in him invented psychoanalysis.

During the time that hypnosis was being invented, several physicians began using hypnosis for anesthesia. Recamier, in 1821 performed an operation while using hypnosis as anesthesia. John Elliotson, a British surgeon in 1834, introduced the stethoscope in England. He reported doing several painless operations by using hypnosis. A Scottish surgeon, James Esdaile, did over 345 major and 2,000 minor operations by using hypnosis during the 1840s and 1850s.

James Braid, a Scottish ophthalmologist, invented modern hypnotism. Braid first used the term nervous sleep or neuro-hypnotism that became hypnosis or hypnotism. Braid went to a demonstration of La Fontaine, the French magnetism in 1841. He ridiculed the Mesmerists' ideas and suggested that hypnosis was psychological. He was the first to practice psychosomatic medicine. He tried to say that hypnosis was just focusing on one idea. Hypnosis was advanced by the Nancy School and is still a term we use today.

The center of hypnosis moved out of Europe and into America. Here it had many breakthroughs in the 20th century. Hypnosis was a popular phenomenon that because more available to normal people who were not doctors. Hypnosis's style changed, too. It was no longer direct instructions from an authority figure instead it became more of a permissive and indirect style of trance that was based on subtle language patterns. This was brought about by Milton H. Erickson. Using hypnosis for quick treatment of trauma and injuries during WWI, WWII, and Korea led to a new interest in hypnosis in psychiatry and dentistry.

Hypnosis started becoming more practical and was thought of as a tool for helping psychological distress. Advances in brain imaging and neurological science along with Ivan Tyrrell and Joe Griffin's work have helped resolve some debates. These British psychologists linked hypnosis to Rapid Eye Movement and brought hypnosis into the realm of daily experiences. The nature of normal consciousness can be understood better as just trance states that we constantly go in and out of.

There are still people who think that hypnosis is a type of power held by the occult even today. The people that believe hypnosis can control minds or perform miracles are sharing the views that have been around for hundreds of years. The history that has been recorded is rich with glimpses of practices and ancient rituals that look like modern hypnosis. The Hindu Vedas have healing passes. An Ancient Egypt has their magical texts. These practices were used for religious ceremonies like communicating with spirits and gods. We need to remember that what people view as the occult was science at its finest in that time frame. It was doing exactly the same thing as modern science was doing now trying to cure human ailments by increasing our knowledge.

Finding the history of hypnosis is like searching for something that is right in our view. We can begin to see it for what it actually is – a phenomenon that is a complicated part of human existence. Hypnosis's future is to completely realize our natural hypnotic abilities and the potential we all hold inside us.

How this book can help you

It does not matter how you feel or what you're suspecting in your body, so long as you see signs that you are losing control of your body weight, then you should be evidence of your physical appearance. Seeing these signs is one thing; understanding what they mean is another thing. This book does not involve practices that you should rush or practices that you should do without a routine and a goal if you mean to change your body weight drastically. Now when it comes to knowing if your body's weight is perfect and if you have full control, then you should make sure that you have used various measures to influence your subconscious mind involved in the practices that will help to keep it in check.

To that end, you will find this book educative, and you will find valuable information meant to keep you as alert as possible in ensuring that you understand how to use this hypnotic gastric band to help to keep your body within the ideal weight and appearance. You will also learn some crucial insights that are related to hypnosis and meditation, and how you can incorporate overeating, powerful affirmations, and visualization aids to achieve your ideal weight and help to improve your relationship with food. Most of the practices that you will carry out might appear impossible, because of the negative thoughts in your subconscious mind

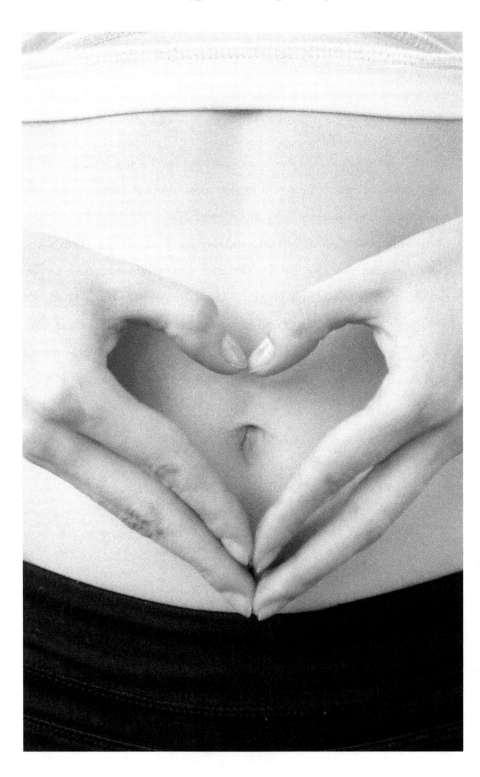

Chapter 1:

Basic of hypnosis and hypnotherapy

What is hypnosis

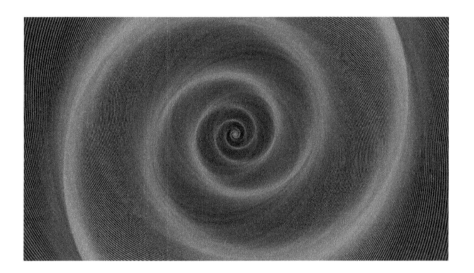

H ypnosis is a state of understanding of focus and concentration. There are two theories about how hypnosis works. The "country" theory implies that subjects enter a different condition of consciousness. The "on-state" concept says that hypnosis isn't an altered state of consciousness. Rather, the topic is responding to a proposal and actively engaging in the semester, Instead of under the control of the hypnotist there are hypnosis methods. Among the very common is that the procedure, which entails keeping a constant stare until the eyes shut at a bright object. You're more when you've entered the state of hypnosis suggestible and more inclined to be more amenable to creating changes. Entering into a trance, relaxed state of consciousness Once a trance, the hypnotist will provide verbal ideas, for example, "if you awaken, you will feel more inspired" or even "you won't drink alcohol." Some argue that hypnosis might help recover repressed memories, treat dependence, cure allergies, and decrease depression and anxiety. Hypnosis is focus and responsiveness to tips. You are inclined to be amenable to creating positive behavioral changes.

What is self hypnosis

The only significant difference between hypnosis and self-hypnosis is that in the first one the operator and the subject are two different people, while in self-hypnosis the operator and the subject coincide in the same person.

It is also a fact that learning is easier and faster when done with another person.

Ask your partner to hypnotize you using a procedure similar to the one we used in the second session. Then practice the self-hypnosis exercise for a few days. Ask your partner once again to hypnotize you and reinforce hypnotic suggestion. Practice it again.

The number of times it is necessary to reinforce the procedure depends entirely on you. If you practice the daily self-hypnosis exercise, one or two reinforcement sessions will be sufficient.

But what about those who have no one with whom to share the learning experience of self-hypnosis? What can they do? How can they learn?

Leave your worries aside.

It is possible to use self-hypnosis to solve virtually any type of problem and also to broaden your consciousness and connect with your innate superior intelligence and creative ability. By using self-hypnosis for the latter purpose, hypnosis can be transformed into a meditation.

Self-hypnosis can also be used in those moments when you feel the need for a higher power to intervene in some situation; Then it becomes a prayer. The subtle differences between these forms of self-hypnosis lies in the way thoughts are guided once the state of consciousness itself has been altered, that is, when the alpha state has been reached.

Then I will tell you a fun experience that happened to me with self-hypnosis. I had an appointment with the dentist to have two molars removed. Last night I had conditioned myself to stop the flow of blood.

The day of the appointment, when sitting in the dentist's chair, I self-reported. When the dentist removed the teeth, I blocked the flow of blood so that it did not flow through the open wound. The dentist was perplexed and kept telling his assistant: «It doesn't bleed.

How is it possible? I don't understand it. I smiled mentally, since I couldn't physically smile because of all the devices, cotton and other objects that held my mouth. In addition, I visualized a quick and complete healing. After seventy-two hours the swelling had subsided, and the wounds had healed completely;

And now I will tell you another funny experience that one of my patients had with self-hypnosis.

He was part of a group that participated in an investigation about dreams at the local hospital. Once a week my patient slept in the hospital with an electroencephalogram (EEG) connected to his head. This was intended to record the waves of their brain activity.

By observing the graph, doctors could establish if they were in alpha, beta, tit or delta state, and they could also state when the patient was sleeping and when he was awake. My client immediately hypnotized himself as soon as he was connected to the EEG.

The apparatus recorded a deep alpha state, indicative that the subject was sleeping, although he was fully awake. One of the doctors asked: "What's going on here?"

Then the man alternately returned to the beta state, then to alpha, then again to beta and finally to alpha while the machine registered it.

The changes confused the doctors until the subject told them what he was doing. The response of the doctors cannot be reproduced here.

What a wonderful tool is self-hypnosis! It transports us to another state while we are comfortably and quietly sitting with our eyes closed thinking about a certain objective. But using self-hypnosis in this sense is not easy to achieve since it requires a prolonged period of preconditioning in a hypnotic or autohypnotic state. Such preconditioning is similar to that used for diet control, but the indications are different; It will be necessary to devise the techniques and suggestions for this case.

And it also requires practice, a lot of practice. Do not forget my words, time and effort will be rewarded with the results. Develop your own discipline and stick to it; The results will be a real success.

History of hypnosis

There are many contradictions in the history of hypnosis. Its history is a bit like trying to find the history of breathing. Hypnosis is a universal trait that was built in at birth. It has been experienced and shared by every human since the beginning of time. It has just been in the past few decades that we are beginning to understand this. Hypnosis hasn't changed in a million years. The way we understand it and how we control it has changed a lot.

Hypnosis has always been surrounded by misconceptions and myths. Despite being used clinically and all the research that has been done, some continue to be scared by the assumption that hypnosis is mystical. Many people think that hypnosis is a modern-day innovation that spread through communities that believed in the metaphysical during the 70s and 80s. Since the mid-1800s, hypnosis was used in the United States. It has advanced with the help of psychologists such as Alfred Binet, Pierre Janet, and Sigmund Freud, and others. Hypnosis can be found in ancient times and has been investigated by modern researchers, physicians, and psychologists.

Hypnosis's origins can't be separated from psychology and western medicine. Most ancient cultures from Roman, Greek, Egyptian, Indian, Chinese, Persian, and Sumerian used hypnosis. In Greece and Egypt, people who were sick would go to the places that healed. These were known as dream temples or sleep temples where people could be cured with hypnosis. The Sanskrit book called "The Law of Manu" described levels of hypnosis such as sleep-walking, dream sleep, and ecstasy sleep in ancient India.

The earliest evidence of hypnosis was found in the Egyptian Ebers Papyrus that dated back to 1550 BC. Priest/physicians repeated suggestions while treating patients. They would have the patient gaze at metal discs and enter a trance. This is now called eye fixation.

During the Middle Ages, princes and kings thought they could heal with the Royal Touch. These healings can be attributed to divine powers. Before people began to understand hypnosis, the terms mesmerism or magnetism would be used to describe this type of healing.

Paracelsus, the Swiss physician, began using magnets to heal. He didn't use a holy relic or divine touch. This type of healing was still being used in the 1700s. A Jesuit priest, Maximillian Hell was famous for healing using magnetic steel plates. Franz Mesmer, an Austrian physician, discovered he could send people into a trance without the use of magnets. He figured out the healing force came from inside himself or an invisible fluid that took up space. He thought that "animal magnetism" could be transferred from the patient to healer by a mysterious etheric fluid. This theory is so wrong. It was based on ideas that were current during the time specifically Isaac Newton's theory of gravity.

Mesmer developed a method for hypnosis that was passed on to his followers. Mesmer would perform inductions by linking his patients together by a rope that the animal magnetism could pass over. He would also wear a cloak and play music on a glass harmonica while all this was happening. The image that a hypnotist was a mystical figure goes back to this.

These practices led to his downfall and for time hypnotism was considered dangerous for anyone to have as a career. The fact remains that hypnosis works. The 19*th* century was full of people who were looking to understand and apply it.

Marquis de Puysegur, a student of Mesmer, was a successful magnetist who first used hypnosis called somnambulism or sleepwalking. Puysegur's followers called themselves experimentalists. Their work recognized that cures didn't come from magnets but an invisible source.

Abbe Faria, an Indo-Portuguese priest, did hypnosis research in India during 1813. He went to Paris and studied hypnosis with Puysegur. He thought that hypnosis or magnetism wasn't what healed but the power that was generated from inside the mind.

His approach was what helped open the psychotherapy hypnosis centered school called Nancy School. The Nancy School said that hypnosis was a phenomenon brought on by the power of suggestion and not from magnetism. This school was founded by a French country doctor, Ambroise-Auguste Liebeault. He was called the father of modern hypnotherapy. He thought hypnosis was psychological and had nothing to do with magnetism. He studied the similar qualities of trance and sleep and noticed that hypnosis was a state that could be brought on my suggestion.

His book **Sleep and Its Analogous States** was printed in 1866. The stories and writings about his cures attracted Hippolyte Bernheim to visit him. Bernheim was a famous neurologist who was skeptical of Liebeault, but once he observed Liebault, he was so intrigued that he gave up internal medicine and became a hypnotherapist. Bernheim brought Liebeault's ideas to the medical world with **Suggestive Therapeutics** that showed hypnosis as a science. Bernheim and Liebeault were the innovators of psychotherapy. Even today, hypnosis is still viewed as a phenomenon.

The pioneers of psychology studied hypnosis in Paris and Nancy Schools. Pierre Janey developed theories of traumatic memory, dissociation, and unconscious processes studied hypnosis with

Bernheim in Charcot in Paris and Nancy. Sigmund Freud studied hypnosis with Charcot and observed both Liebeault and Bernheim. Freud started practicing hypnosis in 1887. Hypnosis was critical in him invented psychoanalysis.

During the time that hypnosis was being invented, several physicians began using hypnosis for anesthesia. Recamier, in 1821 operated while using hypnosis as anesthesia. John Elliotson, a British surgeon in 1834, introduced the stethoscope in England. He reported doing several painless operations by using hypnosis. A Scottish surgeon, James Esdaile, did over 345 major and 2,000 minor operations by using hypnosis during the 1840s and 1850s.

James Braid, a Scottish ophthalmologist, invented modern hypnotism. Braid first used the term nervous sleep or neuro-hypnotism that became hypnosis or hypnotism. Braid went to a demonstration of La Fontaine, the French magnetism in 1841. He ridiculed the Mesmerists' ideas and suggested that hypnosis was psychological. He was the first to practice psychosomatic medicine. He tried to say that hypnosis was just focusing on one idea. Hypnosis was advanced by the Nancy School and is still a term we use today.

The center of hypnosis moved out of Europe and into America. Here it had many breakthroughs in the 20*th* century. Hypnosis was a popular phenomenon that because more available to normal people who were not doctors. Hypnosis's style changed, too. It was no longer direct instructions from an authority figure instead it became more of a permissive and indirect style of trance that was based on subtle language patterns. This was brought about by Milton H. Erickson. Using hypnosis for quick treatment of trauma and injuries during WWI, WWII, and Korea led to a new interest in hypnosis in psychiatry and dentistry.

Hypnosis started becoming more practical and was thought of as a tool for helping psychological distress. Advances in brain imaging and neurological science along with Ivan Tyrrell and Joe Griffin's work have helped resolve some debates. These British psychologists linked hypnosis to Rapid Eye Movement and brought hypnosis into the realm of daily experiences. The nature of normal consciousness can be understood better as just trance states that we constantly go in and out of.

There are still people who think that hypnosis is a type of power held by the occult even today. The people that believe hypnosis can control minds or perform miracles are sharing the views that have been around for hundreds of years. The history that has been recorded is rich with glimpses of practices and ancient rituals that look like modern hypnosis. The Hindu Vedas have healing passes. Ancient Egypt has its magical texts. These practices were used for religious ceremonies like communicating with spirits and gods. We need to remember that what people view as the occult was science at its finest in that time frame. It was doing the same thing as modern science was doing now trying to cure human ailments by increasing our knowledge.

Finding the history of hypnosis is like searching for something that is right in our view. We can begin to see it for what it actually is – a phenomenon that is a complicated part of human existence. Hypnosis's future is to completely realize our natural hypnotic abilities and the potential we all hold inside us.

For so many years now, individuals have been contemplating and contending about this topic. All hypnosis scientists are yet to explain how it really works. With hypnosis, you'll be able to see an individual under a trance, but you won't understand what is going on. This trance is a little piece of how human personality works. It is safe to say that hypnosis will continue to remain a mystery to us. We all know the general aspects of hypnosis, but we can't truly understand how it works. Hypnosis is a condition of series portrayed by serious suggestive expanded and unwinding dreams. It is not sleeping, because when you are under hypnosis, you are still under alert. But you are simply wondering into fantasyland, and you feel yourself going into another dimension that is different from this physical dimension.

You are completely mindful, but you are not mindful of the environment around you. You are only mindful of that thing that is being portrayed in your mind and that dreamland that you are going into. In your normal day of life, you can feel the universe and the universe effect on your feelings. Research has shown that hypnosis can be used to cure several conditions. It is effective in elevating conditions like rheumatism joint pains. It helps to elevate labor pains and childbearing pains. It has also been used to reduce diamante side effects. It also helps in ADHD side effects hypnotherapy. And it reduces the impact of sickness in the body. It also helps during torment. It can also help to improve dental pains and skin conditions like moles.

It also helps to cure disorder manifestation. Also, it can be used to ease the torment of agony brought about by childbirth and childbearing. It also helps to cure smoking, reduce weight, and stop bedwetting.

Where is hypnosis utilized

Through research, spellbinding has been utilized in the treatment of different conditions, for example,

Alleviating constant excruciating conditions like rheumatoid joint pain Alleviating and treating torment in labor

Reducing dementia side effects

For some ADHD side effects, hypnotherapy might be of assistance

Reducing the impacts of sickness prompting retching in disease patients on chemotherapy

Reducing torment when experiencing a dental technique

Improving and taking out skin conditions, for example, psoriasis and moles

Reducing touchy inside disorder manifestations

So, for what reason should an individual endeavor in spellbinding? In certain examples, people might search for entrancing to help constant agony or ease torment and nervousness brought about by restorative procedures, for example, medical procedure or birth.

Mesmerizing has likewise been utilized to help people with conduct changes, for example, smoking end, weight reduction, or bed-wetting counteractive action.

Misconceptions about hypnosis

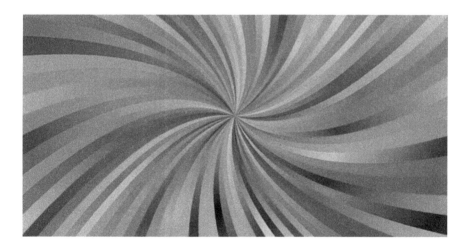

There are too many mistakes regarding hypnosis, many of which have been broadcast by movies that deal with people turned into zombies by an extremely powerful person who exclaims: "Look me in the eye!" This may be interesting, but It is mere fiction and has no relation to the truth. Next we will expose some of the most common myths and explain them. A hypnotist has magical powers . This is absolutely false.

A hypnotist is a normal human being who has prepared to use the power of suggestion in order to cause certain desired results by the hypnotized person.

A person who is hypnotized can do things against his will . Completely false. First, nobody can be hypnotized against their will. It is essential that the subject wishes to cooperate. Secondly, no person who has been hypnotized can be forced to do something they would not do in a normal state. During hypnosis, the subject can accept or reject any suggested order. If what the hypnotist proposes disturbs the subject, in all likelihood he will quickly leave the hypnotic state.

It is only possible to hypnotize people with weak minds . The opposite is true. The smarter a person is, the easier it will be to hypnotize him. In fact, in certain cases of mental weakness it is absolutely impossible to practice hypnosis. It is possible to hypnotize practically all those who wish to be hypnotized. Only 1 percent of the population cannot be hypnotized due to mental deficiencies or other reasons beyond our understanding.

A hypnotized person is in a trance or unconscious . Absolutely fake. A subject undergoing hypnosis is awake and aware: extremely conscious. What happens is that he has simply focused his attention where the hypnotist has indicated and has abstracted himself from everything else.

Anyone can remain in a hypnotic state forever . This is completely false. Even assuming that the hypnotist died after hypnotizing the subject, he would leave the hypnotic state easily, either falling into a short sleep and then waking normally or opening his eyes when he did not hear the hypnotist's voice for a while.

To obtain positive results, a state of deep hypnosis is necessary . Is not true. Any level of hypnosis can offer good results.

HYPNOTIC STATE.-

Any person undergoing hypnosis is very aware of where they are and what is happening. The subject hears everything that happens while immersed in a state similar to daytime sleep, deeply relaxed. He often feels the body numb or has no awareness of having a body.

SELF HYPNOSIS.-

It is possible to self hypnotize. Many people do it daily to give constructive orders. It is much easier to self hypnotize if you have already gone through the experience of having been hypnotized by another person and received the instructions to do so. Through this book you will learn to hypnotize other people but with the same instructions you will learn to self hypnotize. If you work with someone who hypnotizes you, you will accelerate the spread of self hypnosis learning.

Procedures of hypnosis

There are different procedures that you will follow when doing hypnosis. The first one is analytical techniques. That technique is good for unwinding. There are various approaches to start an illogical treatment session. The first session will tend to put you in a comfortable chair and make you close your eyes, and then your specialist will utilize a smooth calming voice and move you down gradually intentionally. He might even put his hand on your chest at certain times. So when undergoing this hypothesis, try to keep the photos of the subject in a great way

Chapter 2:

Hypnosis for weight loss

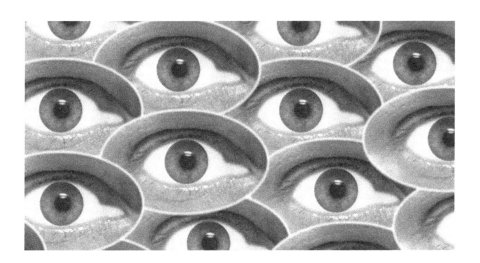

How hypnosis can be used for weight loss

N ow, as I am walking down the beach, I will come to an area with unpleasant bells written by me in the sand. Those labels have been given to me in the past. Those labels are the labels that have held me back in the past from reaching my true capacity and from reaching my true power. I see those labels in the sand, and I begin to use my leg to clean them and use my legs to wash it off and clean the area with sweeping. With my feet, I erase the words away with every stroke of my feet, and I watch as the water comes to the shore to clear them away and clear all this around me.

Those words mean nothing to me; they do not exist again because I was the only one that saw them. I turn them around, and I work a little way down the beach. I feel more confident and taller. I come to the middle of a large rock sitting in the middle of the sand, and on this rock, there is a little pick. I pick it up, and I begin to write all the things that I want about my life. I begin to write all the things that I want about my weight. I am writing all the things that describe me. I am writing that I am confident, I am talented, and I am accomplished. And that I am a good person. I write as many words as possible that describe me.

I write things like positive, attractive, and capable I look at all the words that I have written on this rock and I know that I am a great person. I begin to recall all the moments whereby I felt confident. I think of the time that I felt confident, and I recall those feelings again. I visualize those convenient moments in my life, and what it felt like, what it sounded like, and I then realize what it smells like. I believe this positive moment in my life. I think of the times where I felt confident in my life.

I feel those feelings. I picture those moments again, and I make the colors brighter and more vivid. I feel those feelings of confidence and pride, and I turn off the sounds and the smells. I get back into those moments where I was feeling so confident and powerful that I was feeling so confident in myself and all the things that I was doing. I am confident in the way I look. I am confident in the way I dress, and I'm confident in the way I act. I am confident in my relationship. I am confident in the relationship that I have with the members of the opposite sex. I am confident in the relationship that I have with my family with my friends and my coworkers.

Things come to me easily, with the way I talk to people. Conversations come out fluently from my mouth, and people respect what I have to say. I am strong and respected, and everyone around me sees me as confident and capable I take a look at myself, and I see that I am full of positive energy. I am the one that is radiating how everyone sees me. Everyone around me sees the positive energy in me, not only the people around me, but I also respect myself. I stand tall and strong. I stand proud of myself. I know that I can accomplish whatever I put my mind to accomplish. All I am seeing are positive things in my life.

I have practical and creative ideas, and I fill my mind with positive energy. I drop the future and go forward with confidence. I imagine myself one year from now, and I imagine the person that I will grow up to be. When I imagine this image, I will not be able to recognize the person that I once was. I have accomplished great things in the past year, great things that will help me to reach my capabilities.

My confidence has enabled others to look at me with great confidence and respect. I enjoy talking with people, and they're interested in what I have to say. My career is going great, and I can voice my ideas and opinions to other people because they value them. The relationship with my friends and families are great. Most of my friends and families come to seek advice from me because they hold me in high esteem. I look at myself, and I see how positive I am. I can point others in the right direction that they should go. I have faith in myself. I have great ideas, and I know that my family and friends respect my ideas, and they know my values too. I hold my head high and I know that nothing can bring me down. I stand tall and strong because I know that I am an accomplished, beautiful, capable and confident person.

Hypnosis and eating habits

There are multiple types of diets or nutritional options, such as Paleolithic diet, autoimmune diet, GAPS diet, Okinawa diet, food guide according to the study of China, Mediterranean diet, intermittent fasting, ketogenic diet, detox diet, Montignac diet, diet Dunkan, Atkins diet, macrobiotic diet, vegetarian diet, vegan diet, and so on.

Some of the diets are supported by the official scientific community and others are not. However, from my point of view and experience, all are valid depending on each person, moment and circumstance. In addition, we all have much to discover, including the official scientific community.

All diets or eating guides have something in common, which is to restrict food to improve digestion. And by improving digestion, more nutrients are obtained with less effort. The function of our digestive system is optimized, and health is improved. On the planet, energy is neither created nor destroyed, it simply transforms. And our digestive system transforms the energy of food into useful energy for our body .

Consuming less quantity, as long as it allows us to reach the energy we need, means being more sustainable with the environment and with our body. Our body becomes more efficient in all its functions, and stays healthier and younger. And the same goes for the planet.

BUT HOW DO YOU GET TO EAT A SMALL AMOUNT, FEEL SATIATED, BE NOURISHED AND HAVE ENERGY?

Success is based on the perfect combination and processing of food. That is, balance macronutrients and boost micronutrients. The components of the food and drink we consume interact with each other. Knowing how to process and combine them correctly, we improve digestion and maximize their bioavailability. This will bring us enormous benefits for our health (better nutrition) and for the planet (better use of resources). AN EXAMPLE IS AS FOLLOWS:

Kale, strawberries, corn, eggs, black garlic, and olive oil Balance the macronutrients of each meal. For example, according to the healthy dish of the example, for an adult: 2 boiled eggs (animal protein has greater bioavailability), 200 gr. Sweet corn (carbohydrates: starch and sugar), 100 gr. of kale (curly cabbage) massaged with olive oil (healthy fats) and strawberries (vitamins, minerals, and fiber).

Combine micronutrients to improve digestion and enhance its nutritional value. For example: green leafy vegetables with healthy fats. Green leafy vegetables help digest fats, and fats help absorb vitamins from vegetables. Save work for the intestine, eating predigested food. As for example: crushed,marinated, massaged, fermented vegetables;

yogurt; dextrinated bread; hot proteins; natural sweet food. Distinguish between physiological and emotional hunger. And eat only in the presence of the first.

How to use self – hypnosis

There are several self-hypnosis techniques out there; however, they are all based on one concept: focusing on a single idea, object, image, or word. This is the key that opens the door to trance. You can achieve focus in many ways, which is the reason why there are so many different techniques that can be applied. After a period of initial learning, those who have learned a method, and have continued to practice it, realize that they can skip certain steps. In this part, we will take a look at the essential self-hypnosis techniques.

What is a self-hypnosis session

Now we will go over 10 simple and succinct steps to perform a successful and fruitful and positively effective session of self-hypnosis. I will list the steps first and follow up with a step-by-step breakdown featuring a brief and easy to understand the description of what each step should entail for you in your journey.

Step 1: Preparation of Self

Step 2: Preparation of Time

Step 3: Preparation of Space

Step 4: Preparation of Goal and Motive

Step 5: Relaxation of the Physical Body

Step 6: Relaxation of the Soul and the Mind

Step 7: Realization of Trance

Step 8: Active Repetition of Mantra or Performance of Script

Step 9: Preparation for Exiting the Trance State

Step 10: Returning to Earth

As you read those steps, I'm sure they bring forth images in your mind. It may seem apparent already what you have to do, and ideas for how to guide yourself through this self-hypnosis you are preparing for are blossoming like wildfire in your mind. Let us go more in-depth, to further prepare and become aware of all that you can do to make your self-hypnosis as easy and effective as your soul will wish, to better yourself in the most transformative way possible.

Step 1: Preparation of Self

So, as you are aware, one of the first and foremost goals is to become as relaxed as possible, before, during, and after entering the trance-state. Relaxation is the key that helps us enter the trance-state, and the trance-state further facilitates relaxation of the entire being both during the active self-hypnosis and afterward, for positive benefits of your being. To achieve the most successful self-hypnosis possible, we must first prepare ourselves, our minds and our physical bodies, for what we desire to achieve, a state of heightened relaxation in which we can become hyper-aware of the inner machinations of the mind, to achieve a closer union with them, to bond with them, and to converse with them on the most intimate level possible. This can mean many things to many people. Go to the used CD store, and you will see an endless section of new age music, monks chanting, flute playing, choirs, and tribal drums. The popularity of this music exists because people desire for sounds that will lull them into a more peaceful state. Maybe you would like to try something like this. Some people prefer silence; some people prefer peaceful noise; a sort of hypnotizing drone that guides them into a more relaxed state of being. White noise, be it from a fan, a laundry machine, running water, or a white noise machine made specifically for the purpose of filling the air with a light white noise, can also be effective for this purpose. Anything that has the desired effect on you will serve this purpose. Another thing, you can do is to drink a nice herbal tea of your choosing; find a blend that is relaxing to you as an individual. Some common choices would be lavender-orange teas or chamomile teas. These will set a space internally for you to prepare yourself for entering your trance-state. Another very common tool for the preparation of the self for self-hypnosis is aromatherapy. Many essential oils, either applied directly to the body or dispersed through the air with the use of an essential oil diffuser, readily and commonly available at most grocery stores, can have a very relaxing effect on the mind and body, ideal for the preparation of self-hypnosis.

Many essential oil manufactures make and sell blends specifically for the purposes of relaxation or stress-relief. Any of these would be a very good choice for a consumer who is feeling anxious about the large selection of essential oils to choose from and would like some advice on which to get. For those who would prefer to buy oils individually, some common choices for the purposes of relaxation would be, again, lavender, a go-to for many people in many situations, clay sage, ylang-ylang, lemon, or jasmine. Most importantly, find a way to put yourself in a good mood and prepare yourself for an inner-journey. Know that many different things work for many different people, and these are all just suggestions. Find what works for you and find your inner peace.

Step 2: Preparation of Time

It goes without saying that if an alarm clock goes on when you are in your trance-state, the effectiveness of your self-hypnosis session will be largely inhibited. It is necessary, if you wish for an effective and transformative session of self-hypnosis, that you make sure a certain amount of time is allotted where you will be safe, secure, at peace, and uninterrupted by your daily responsibilities. Many things can get in the way of this. Common inhibitors of time include children, chores, spouses, day-to-day noise, and work. If you have children, maybe you can have a relative or a reliable babysitter, watch them for a certain amount of time. Maybe you could ask your spouse to take the children out for an hour or two and explain to them your intentions of performing a transformative inner-journey that requires the utmost relaxation possible. If your children are of the age where they go to school, maybe you could find the time while they are away at school. There are many possibilities, but they require planning and foresight to make sure you have your time to do what you need to do to achieve what you plan to achieve through the designated self-hypnosis session. Spouses or other life partners are much easier to deal with as, unlike children, who require constant attention and care, spouses can have the situation explained to them and are generally ready and willing to give you any space you will need to do anything that you feel will make yourself happier and more at peace. If you are in an honest and communicative relationship, they should already be well on your side as far as your self-hypnosis journey is concerned. Day-to-day noise is something that can be accounted for if it is an issue. If you are living in a place where certain times of the day have excessive traffic outside or nearby, either driving traffic or foot traffic, just keep that in mind when allotting time for your self-hypnosis. If you live across the street from a public school, do not plan your self-hypnosis journey when it is just about time for school to get out, as you will be interrupted by and inundated with an unwelcome rush of noise, and possibly loud bells signaling the end of the day. And, lastly, work should be no issue. If work follows you home, by a cell-phone linked to a work line or other such method, send it straight to voice mail for a time, let whoever is in charge know that you are in need of private time and will be away from the line shortly. These things can always be worked out with whomever they need to be worked out with. Responsibilities can be many and growing and overwhelming. Situations in which you have a large burden of responsibility ironically are the types of situations that can make necessary long and fruitful journeys into self-hypnosis. It takes planning and care to make sure that, while all responsibilities are met, there is a designated and a specified time for you to go into your journey with the utmost confidence and care that you will be able to do what you need to do, and come out the other end as enlightened as possible.

Step 3: Preparation of Space

It also should go without saying that a crowded, busy subway station at peak times of the day is no place for you to go about your most effective journeys into self-hypnosis or the trance-like state. Place is of the essence. Just as your body temple must be totally clean and prepped and ready for the ascension, so must your surrounding area be prepared for you to feel as comfortable as possible to allow for the most successful transition into a strong and malleable trance-like state, allowing for the most successful self-hypnosis possible. Depending on your living situation, this one may or may not be so simple. A young man or woman who is living with several roommates to get by might have a hard time finding a place where they can be alone for a certain amount of time, allowing for the relaxation required to fulfill the depths of the trance. It is up to you, both subject and practitioner, to find where you are most comfortable, and make that space available during the time you have allotted for your self-hypnosis session. You have the freedom to get as creative as you wish. Obviously, for those of you who have homes and places where you are able to spend as much personal time with yourself as you could possibly desire, this task will be the easiest. For others, it can involve hiking to a secluded place, going to a library or other place where silence is golden, a public park at a low-trafficked time of day when few people are there, or even renting a motel or hotel room for a specific amount of time. Do what is necessary so you can perform the actions necessary to better yourself. Once a space is found, the task moves to the setting or dressing of the space. Find a position where you are comfortable, using whatever tools or accessories are required to make yourself as relaxed as possible— blankets, pillows, tranquil pictures or statues such as of deities, indoor waterfalls or fountains, zen gardens, rocks, crystals, orgone generators, the aforementioned essential oil diffusers or white noise machines, any external item that will set the scene for your inner-journey. As always, it is different for different people, depending on beliefs, religion, and personal comforts. Feel free to experiment and find what makes you most comfortable. No one knows how to make you as comfortable as possible, like yourself. Trusting yourself is both one of the biggest keys and one of the biggest goals of self-hypnosis in general, so you must trust yourself here.

Step 4: Preparation of Goal and Motive

One of the critical factors of self-hypnosis is having a plan for what specific change or changes you wish to enact once having entered the trance state, and how you plan to achieve them. This is where the narratives you wish to express, the prayers, or the mantra or mantras you wish to repeat to yourself, come into play. What do you hope to achieve in your self-hypnosis session? It is always different for different people and at different times. But there is always at least one goal, and preparation for achieving that goal is a must when it comes to performing a successful and fruitful and transformative self-hypnosis session. Imagine you are about to have a very important conversation with a very important person in your life. There is something you really need to tell them, and it is of the utmost importance that this conversation goes well and is effective. You will likely have a plan for what you want to say and how you are going to say it. The absolute same thing goes here, where you are about to have a very deep and meaningful conversation with the self. You must know what you are going to tell yourself, and how you are going to say it. Therefore, you must be totally aware of your goal, what you wish to achieve through the act of self-hypnosis. It is imperative that you don't try to fix everything wrong with your entire life at once, you must be focused, and you must be honed in on one specific, changeable thing at a time. The rest will come later. You are crossing a river one stepping stone at a time, putting one foot in front of the other, and you will make it across if you stay steady, attentive, and aware of your surroundings. Be calm, be collected, and be prepared for what you are about to do.

Step 5: Relaxation of the Physical Body

Now we begin. There are many schools of thought on the best ways to relax the body. One very common through-line in all of these is the act of deep, conscious breathing. Breath in, breath out, be aware of your breaths, be in control of each one of them. The goal here is mainly to become aware of every single voluntary and involuntary action of the physical body and slow it down. Feel your heartbeat. Be aware of it. Envision it slowing down. Relax. Expand the space and the length of each breath. Focus on certain areas of the body and watch them become more and more still.

For you, I will share my personal method. First, I put my awareness into my feet. I breathe in and hold my awareness in my feet, then I exhale and feel my feet get heavier and lighter at the same time. Repeat this process about 10 times, and it will feel as if your feet have left your body, having floated away down a stream of serenity. Now work up. Do this for every section of your body, all the way up to your head. Now you will feel totally weightless, as if you are suspended in midair, effortlessly. Your awareness now becomes of your entire physical being, holistically. You are aware of no specific part of yourself but your entirety. Float down the river. The deep breaths will have become unconscious, the world and your body have achieved a kind of totally unthinking symbiosis. Each breath sustains and gives power to the relaxed state. Your whole body is more relaxed than you have ever felt it; it is supernatural and, for some, can be kind of intimidating. There are places you can go that you have never been to before, and you can go there without ever leaving the house. Cherish the feeling, and follow it out the door. Now that you have achieved a state of total physical relaxation, you are totally, still, unmoving, and there is nothing but you and your mind. Let us proceed to relax the mind as we have the body.

Step 6: Relaxation of the Soul and the Mind

So to relax the mind, we can perform a series of steps very similar to those shown when relaxing the body but carried over to another plane. Just as in relaxing the physical body our goal was to become totally aware of all voluntary and involuntary actions of the body, so as to slow them down to a point where they are more malleable and understandable, so too here, we must become aware of all the voluntary and involuntary actions of the mind, so as to slow them down to a point where they are more malleable and understandable. It is like slowly zooming in with a microscope, so things that were once small, almost imperceptible, become very large and monolithic. Our goal is to achieve a state of hyper-awareness.

I eschewed the act of visualization from the previous step, although visualization can play a vital role in either step because I feel it is most pertinent here in this step.

Visualization, as we know, is primarily mental and therefore, most effective and necessary in the mental landscape. It is the mental landscape where we see images and things that we know do not exist in the physical world before us. They exist through the power of and only inside of our imagination. Anything can exist there, and it is the realm where we are the ultimate creators of anything we desire. It goes without saying, the things we conjure up in our imagination may not appear before us instantly, manifested by our mere thought but they do have an extreme and very palpable effect on our physical reality, an effect which the act of self-hypnosis aims to hone and control. So we will explore means of visualization and the effect that this can have upon us as we aim to enter that state of trance necessary for self-hypnosis.

You may or may not have become in your life familiar with guided meditations, where someone, be it a speaker in your vicinity or someone on a CD or audiotape, or even a YouTube video or MP3, recites a narrative that you put yourself in mentally with the intention of guiding yourself into a more peaceful state of being. They will often say things like "Imagine that you are weightless," or "Imagine that you are floating in space," or "Imagine that you are witnessing the most serene sunset in the most beautiful location possible with the love of your life." The key is to imagine yourself either being something that is more relaxed than you are now or being in a time or place, derived from fantasy or personal memory, that facilitates the transition into a more relaxed state than you are in now. You can imagine a time and place when or where you felt as free as you ever have in your life. A loved one who passed away, who you found comfort with as a child, you can imagine they are there with you, in another dimension, feeding you the love you remember. You can imagine that you are flying, effortlessly, through the cosmos. Totally uninhibited, feeling a sense of freedom hitherto unfelt. You can imagine that you are floating in the ocean, totally unattached to anything resembling typical human constructs or society. Your imagination is your own personal canvas, and here you are, free to paint any picture you can imagine. Imagining specific senses and perceptions, especially when your body is hyper-relaxed, can lead to both ecstatic levels of mental peace and real feelings of the senses that you are experiencing what you imagine. This is a tool with unlimited power in the act and journey of self-hypnosis.

Step 7: Realization of Trance

Now you are here, and you have willfully affected the realization of the trance-like state that is the initial aim of a good, effective session of proper self-hypnosis. Let your awareness span out through the eternity of reality as it is, allow your entire being the freedom to seep out through the full bounds of this new state, float there where you are and simply exist for a time as you marvel in the state you have achieved. With or without the added benefit of the active involvement of your will for the specific and guided change that defines self-hypnosis, this state of being you have entered into is medicinal and a very pure, enlightening experience to be in. So be in it. Float, again, down the river. Float down the river of the self, float down the river of life, float down the river of the universe. For a time, allow yourself just to feel what it is to be an inactive agent in the cosmos. Step outside of yourself, float above yourself, and look back, or down, or beside, and see who you are. Does it look familiar? Know yourself. Know yourself, here, and now, as you have never known yourself before. Feel the intimacy you have achieved with yourself. Feel intimate feelings that you may have never felt before, for anyone, yourself or others. This is you. Don't be afraid to reach out and touch the light. Fully immerse yourself in this experience that you have prepared for. Know that you are achieving a very important and personal goal, and be glad and grateful and ecstatic and proud about where you are. Feel the ball of light at your core, your solar plexus, emanating out like a shining star, like the sun, like the soil. It may be orgasmic. You may be taken aback by the power you have tapped into, the infinite potential. Focus on the awareness of the self and see who you are.

Step 8: Active Repetition of Mantra or Performance of Script

Now you have journeyed into space. Speak. Your voice echoes into the cosmos with a power you have never felt. You have never heard your voice this loud and powerful and confident. It is incredible. The memories you are creating here, of your own voice, are going to be some of the most powerful memories you've ever had, totally overriding any past traumatic experience, any other voices, the outliers, the negative drones. These were all nothing. This is everything. Even very simple sounds begin to take on their own gravitational pull that is so large. You are the sun, and you are creating planets to orbit you with each word spoken. It is the inner-voice, in preparation for the inner-dialogue. We are about to do it.

Speak the words you wish to speak to yourself. Each repetition of the mantra will completely change the landscape that you have found yourself in seismic waves. You will feel a growing energy completely under your control swarm over your entire being and beyond. You are in charge here. What you say goes. You are the ruler of this land, and you are going to take care of it well and make sure it is a prosperous paradise. Watch the negative thoughts, the images, the shadows, the memories you feared, the people you hate, the guilt, the pain, watch it shrivel into dust and evaporate before your very eyes, melted into oblivion by the sheer overwhelming power you have achieved.

Step 9: Preparation for Exiting the Trance State

Just as when you fully submersed, take a moment after you are done with your action to appreciate the beauty of what you are witnessing. Just be here now in this state. It is an eternal state. You will leave, and you will go back to the physical world, but this state will stay, untouched, eternal, waiting for you to return. This is heaven. Know that you are about to return, and you are about to feel very different than you have ever felt before. Embrace these differences. It may be odd and imperfect at first, but it is a learning experience. The physical reality still awaits you as always— a different eternal experience. The rest of your life will be spent juxtaposing these two very different and very real planes and finding the perfect balance where you are in absolute control, yet in total surrender and synchronicity.

Are you ready? You may wish to take one last look around, soak it all in, but eventually, you must prepare for the journey home. It can be as simple as opening your eyes. It might be something that you don't want to do so you better prepare. Step 10: Returning to Earth

Open your eyes. Where are you? Who are you? You may feel like this is something equally new as the realm you have just left. But there is a feeling of familiarity. You are awakened to the infinite possibilities of life. You see that your perspective can change in infinite ways, and with that change in perspective leads a portal to infinite different realties experienced through the multi-faceted crystal that is existence. You may be stunned. You will be changed.

Don't get too excited. Don't run into the other room screaming at your spouse, "I've found the meaning of life! " This is something just for you. Keep it quiet and sacred. Other people will come when they are ready. Your job is simply to exist— at peace.

Maybe you'll want to make some different choices tomorrow, after a nice sleep, an unconscious refresher to the land of dreams, a place that might seem more familiar and close to you than it ever has before. Maybe tomorrow, while you're on your commute to work, you'll spontaneously hear the loud booming voice of God pouring through your brain, reciting that mantra you envisioned for yourself. It's a memory— a memory you have now; a memory you created. It will feel fantastic, and you will feel more in control of your life than you ever have before.

Chapter 3:
Hypnosis portion control

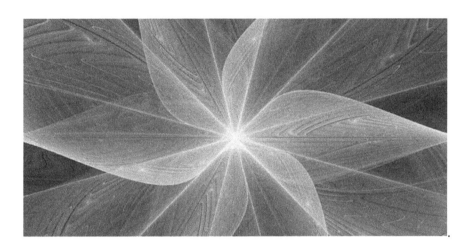

ortion control tends to be a skill that many people struggle with. Knowing how to eat just enough to help yourself feel satisfied and full, without overeating, can be challenging. This is made even more challenging if you tend to be a stress eater or someone who goes long periods of time without eating and then binge eats.

Portion control is an incredibly important element of weight loss as it provides you with the opportunity to get the proper nutrients into your body without overdoing it. As well, if you choose to satisfy one of your cravings or enjoy something more indulgent, portion control enables you to do so without going overboard.

The truth is: most people can eat anything in moderation and not suffer any unwanted consequences from eating that food. For example, if you want to enjoy a piece of brownie with your coffee at the café because you have been craving a brownie, there is typically nothing wrong with doing that.

The key is to make sure that you enjoy the brownie, and then you stop. Rather than enjoying that brownie, then eating another piece, then going home and having even more junk food, enjoy that one brownie and then let yourself get back on track with healthy eating. When you can mindfully engage in portion control this way, you can eat just about anything you want without having any problems.

In fact, many famous diets rely more on portion control than anything else because they recognize that portion control is more effective than restricting what people can and cannot eat.

The key with portion control is knowing how to actually feel satisfied by your controlled portions and knowing how to stay committed to them. For many people, this can be challenging. You may feel so happy about eating your brownie or your piece of cake that you want more immediately after. Of course, if you immediately indulge, then you are not effectively engaging in portion control.

However, if you instead let yourself enjoy that piece as much as you possibly can and then go back to eating healthy immediately after, then there was no big deal.

Rather than relying solely on portion control as a tool, it is important that you rewire your mind around why you struggle with portion control as it is. Getting to the root cause of your own struggles with portion control, healing your overeating challenges, and rewiring your mind around portion control can be incredibly helpful in allowing you to get what you need out of your diet.

This way, rather than dealing with that internal conflict around, "I should stop," you stop naturally because your mind is already wired to stop naturally. As you might suspect, this can be done with subconscious work and hypnosis. However, there are also some conscious-level changes that you should make and things you should become mindful of so that you can navigate portion control both with your conscious mind and your new subconscious habits. This way, you are more likely to be successful with portion control in general.

What is overeating

Overeating is a disorder characterized by a compulsive diet that prevents people from losing control and being unable to stop eating. Final episodes last 30 minutes or work intermittently throughout the day.

An excess dining room will eat without stopping or paying attention to what you eat, even if you are already bored. Overeating can make you feel sick, guilty, and out of control. If you want to know how to stop overeating, follow these steps:

MAINTAINING MENTAL STRENGTH

Stress managing stress is the most frequent cause of overeating. Regardless of whether you are aware or not, the chance is to make a fuss because you are worried about other aspects of your life, such as work, personal relationships, and the health of loved ones.

The easiest way to reduce compulsive intake is to manage life stress. This is a solution that cannot be achieved with a tip bag that can help with stressful situations.

Think about: are there some factors that are stressing your life? How can these factors be minimized? For example, if you are living with an unbearable roommate that is one of the leading causes of stress in your life, it may be time to get out of that situation.

Activities such as yoga, meditation, long walks, listening to jazz and classical music can be enjoyed comfortably. Do what you have to do to feel that you are in control of your life. Try to go to bed at the same time every day and get enough rest. If you are well-rested, you will be better able to cope with stressful situations.

PERFORM AN EXERCISE ROUTINE THAT YOU LIKE

Exercise not only will make you feel healthier, but it will also improve your mental health and make you feel more in control of your body. The trick to exercise is to do something you like instead of feeling that you are using to compensate for binge eating.

Exercise should feel like fun, not torture. Do not do anything you hate. If you hate running, walking or hiking, look for a new activity, such as salsa dancing, Pilates or volleyball. You will have fun doing something you like and you will get more health in the process. Find a gym or exercise with a friend. Having a friend who works with you will make your training more fun and make you feel more motivated.

AVOID TEMPTATION

Another way to avoid overeating is to stay away from situations that can lead to committing them. Taking steps to prevent overeating when you leave home has a significant impact on how you handle your cravings. Avoiding temptation means recognizing a high-risk situation and creating a plan to avoid it. This is what you should do:

Try to spend more time on social activities that do not eat food. Take a walk or walk with friends, or meet friends at a bar that you know is not serving meals. If you are going to a family party that you know will be full of delicious food and desserts, choose a low calorie or healthy option.

Try to escape from unhealthy food when you are at a party. Modify the routine as needed. Eliminate or save a little bit of unhealthy food at home. I don't want to remove all unhealthy snacks from home and go to the stores they sell at midnight.

MANAGING SOCIAL MEALS

When eating out, it is natural to increase the tendency to release because you feel less controlled than the environment and normal diet options. However, being outside should not be an excuse to enjoy overeating.

You must also find ways to avoid them, even if you are in a social environment or surrounded by delicious food. Method is as follows.

Snack before departure. By eating half of the fruit and soup, you can reduce your appetite when surrounded by food. If you are in an area with unlimited snacks, close your hands.

Hold a cup or a small plate of vegetables to avoid eating other foods. If you are in a restaurant, check the menu for healthier options. Try not to be influenced by your friends. Also, if you have a big problem with bread consumption, learn to say "Don't add bread" or smoke peppermint candy until you have a meal.

TAKE TIME TO LISTEN TO THE BODY AND CONNECT THE MIND AND BODY.

If you know what your body is telling you, it will be easier for you to understand what will bring you to your anger and manage your diet. Listen to your body throughout the day and give it time to have a better idea about what it needs or wants.

Follow the 10-minute rule before eating a snack. If you have a desire, do not grant yourself immediately, wait 10 minutes, and look back at what is happening. Ask yourself whether you are hungry or craving. If you are hungry, you have to eat something before your desire grows.

If you have a strong desire but are tired, you must find a way to deal with that feeling. For example, take a walk or do something else to distract from your desires. Ask yourself whether you are eating just because you are bored.

Are you looking in the fridge just because you are looking for something? In that case, find a way to keep yourself active by drinking a glass of water. Please have fun from time to time.

If you have the all-purpose desire to eat peanut butter, eat a spoonful of butter with a banana. This will allow you to reach the breakpoint after 5 days and not eat the entire peanut butter jar.

Maintain healthy habits Eat healthy meals three times a day. This is the easiest way to avoid overeating. If you haven't eaten for half a day, you'll enjoy the fuss. The important thing is to find a way to eat the healthy food you like.

So instead of eating what you want, you feel that you are fulfilling your duty through a dull and tasteless meal, your meal should be nutritious and delicious.

The method is as follows.

Always eat in the kitchen or another designated location. Do not eat even in front of a TV or computer or even when you are on the phone. There is less opportunity to enjoy without concentrating on what you eat. Eat at least 20-25 minutes with each meal.

This may seem like a long time, but it prevents you from feeling when your body is full. There is a gap between the moment your body is full and the moment you feel full, so if you bite a bit more time, you will be more aware of how much you eat.

Each meal needs a beginning and an end. Do not bob for 20 minutes while you cook dinner. Also, do not eat snacks while making healthy snacks. You need to eat three types of food, but you should avoid snacking between meals, avoiding healthy options such as fruits, nuts, and vegetables.

Eat meals and snacks in small dishes using small forks and spoons. Small plates and bowls make you feel as if you are eating more food, and small forks and spoons give you more time to digest the food.

CONNECT YOUR MIND AND BODY OVERTIME

You can get more out of your feelings by writing a diary that lets you write what you have come up with, talk about your desires, and look back after an overwhelming episode.

Taking a little time a day to think about your actions and feelings can have a huge impact on how you approach your life.

Be honest with yourself. Write about how you feel about every aspect of life and your relationship with food.

You can surprise yourself too. You can keep a record of the food you eat unless you are obsessed with every little thing you eat. Sometimes you can escape temptation if you know that you have to write everything you eat.

Hypnosis session for portion control

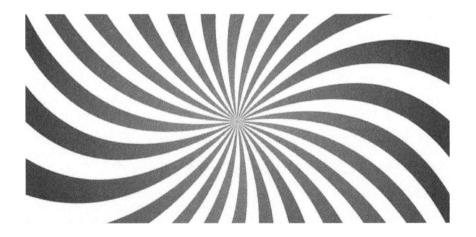

Portion control can assume a noteworthy job in achieving your objectives for wellbeing and weight. You may, as of now, eat all the right sustenance and practice appropriately. In any case, in case regardless you're conveying overabundance weight, it may be because you're simply expending excessively. Control of segments can make a huge distinction.

Great portion control won't just thin you down, it will give you more vitality. Eating the right amount will suggest that your body needs to work more enthusiastically to process superfluous surplus nourishment.

With regards to getting your eating regimen right and shedding surplus fat, the amount is as fundamental as quality. If you have to get thinner, a lot of a decent thing can truly be terrible for you. However, knowing how, when, and the amount to cut so you can truly begin seeing some improvement in accomplishing your weight targets can be troublesome.

Why Is Portion Control So Hard To Achieve?

Propensity controls our lives substantially more than we understand. We eat because it's an ideal opportunity to eat (even though you had a nibble simply 30 minutes prior).

We're gorging out of good manners, or not having any desire to' squander' what's on our plate, or because we're so used to being full that we've overlooked how to perceive when we've had enough.

Some good judgment things can enable you to control the size of the bit:

You can eat all the more gradually intentionally. This offers your stomach the chance to enlist its totality in your cerebrum and mood killer your hunger.

You can begin your supper with soup-it very well may be fulfilling to have a low-calorie soup and enable you to feel cheerful for your fundamental course with a lot of littler part.

You can utilize the old stunt of the littler plate-so you need to eat littler segments truly.

You can stay away from smorgasbords.

Elements of a Hypnosis Session

Hypnosis Patter

Patter simply means **prepared words** in a hypnosis suggestion or script. "Relaxing more and more with every gentle breath you exhale" is hypnosis patter.

Hypnosis Pre-talk

A conversation with clients where we help them understand what hypnosis really is and eliminate common myths about hypnosis. The second chapter of this book on hypnosis could be considered a hypnosis pre-talk, in written form, yet it's more in-depth for readers who are considering becoming professional hypnotists. This is usually done only once with each client.

One of our primary jobs as hypnotists, is to help our clients remove resistance to change, and be willing to get rid of the elements that caused them issue to begin with.

The hypnosis pre-talk helps to eliminate resistance to change, and resistance to doing hypnosis.

Pre-Hypnosis Interview

A conversation with clients prior to every hypnosis session where we discuss their desired outcomes, results for the week, and anything else pertinent to our work together. This happens every session.

Hypnosis Induction

A technique including hypnosis patter where clients enter into a state of hypnosis. Not all hypnosis inductions are created equal, and it's important to have at least one hypnosis induction that works in minutes and brings your clients to the desired level of hypnotic depth. However, you also do not need dozens of hypnotic inductions either. A few highly effective inductions are preferred for the professional hypnotist.

Testing and Convincing

A professional hypnotist will test clients for hypnotic depth, and once that is complete, will use specific hypnotic phenomena to convince clients that they are in hypnosis. This will deepen their hypnotic state.

Hypnosis Insight Work

Insight work is done while in a deep state of hypnosis to bring clients relief. Insight work includes: Age Regression and Progression, Forgiveness Work, Parts Mediation Work, as well as other powerful perspective shifting techniques that brings our client instantaneous and lasting relief.

Direct Suggestion

Direct suggestion, or hypnotic suggestion, is what most people think of when they think of hypnosis. A direct hypnosis suggestion is directly suggesting something to your clients that will help them achieve their desired result. For example, a direct suggestion for someone wanting to lose weight would be "You only eat when you are actually hungry, and the pounds melt away easier than ever before," and for someone wanting to increase their confidence "You think more clearly, speak more easily, and feel confident in your ability to do whatever it is you want to do in your life with grace and ease."

Direct suggestions are important and powerful, and they are still a part of modern hypnosis – however they have a tendency to fade if not reinforced. The preferred method is to use both insight-based techniques, along with Direct Suggestion for lasting benefit.

Emerging from Hypnosis

Emerging the client includes using hypnosis patter to guide the client from a state of hypnosis back to their normal level of consciousness.

Post-Hypnosis Interview

A conversation after the hypnosis session to reinforce insight gained during the hypnosis process and answer any questions from the client.

Hypnosis session for binge eating

Understanding your own binge eating habits is important, as this allows you to develop a conscious awareness and a sense of mindfulness around why you are binge eating in the first place. When you are able to understand why you binge eat,resolving the root cause of your binge eating becomes easier because you know what to look for and what to be aware of.

Getting to the root cause of your own binge eating can be done by reflecting on your own binge eating cycles and, if necessary, tracking your binge eating cycles so that you can start to identify any possible patterns that exist around your binge eating behaviors. You can easily do this by keeping a food diary, which is a journal where you log everything you have eaten in a day.

Make sure that you write down the time that you ate, what you ate, and how much you ate. Track everything, including little snacks in between.

They may not seem significant, but you might be surprised to see how they add up and what comes of those snacks. Often, people find that they are unaware of how problematic their snacking has actually become until they begin to track it.

As you begin looking for the root cause of your binge eating, you might find that there are actually a few root causes. Often, however, most binge eating patterns can be traced back to one "major" root problem that seems to create more problems than the rest. For example, you might find that you have poor eating habits and often find yourself craving low-quality food, but you might realize that this largely stems from you being an emotional eater.

Or, you might find that you are an emotional eater because you have poor eating problems and so you realize that, during a moment of stress, eating is one thing you can take care of while everything else might seem out of your control.

It is important that you take the time to identify every single root cause of your binge eating and not just the one that stands out the most.

If you are going to have the biggest impact on changing your binge eating patterns, you are going to need to know everything that contributes to your binge eating so that you can be mindful of what might be triggering this behavior.

If you do not focus on and heal all of your root causes for binge eating, you might find yourself binge eating out of habit and justifying it by different root causes every single time. The more thorough you can be with healing this, the more effective you will be, too.

With that being said, you may find it to be particularly overwhelming to attempt to actually resolve all of your root causes at once, especially if you have a few. If it does feel overwhelming, you can focus instead on just dealing with the biggest one and then healing one root cause at a time.

This way, you can make a significant impact on healing your binge eating problems, but you are still able to remain mindful and aware of your other binge eating triggers.

Chapter 4:

Guided hypnosis for weight loss

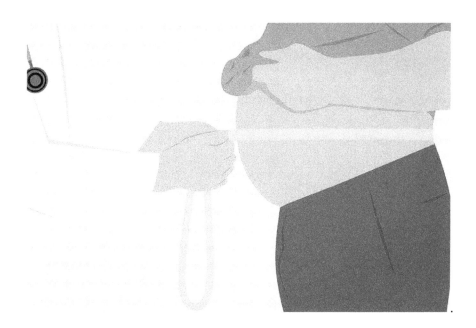

Choosing a hypnotherapist

Expanding open, GP, and NHS acknowledgment of integral treatments and hypnotherapy specifically has brought about a gigantic increment in the number of individuals offering to prepare. The nature of this preparation fluctuates incredibly, so it is the BSCH's main goal to give its specialists an abnormal state of preparing and moral practice.

There are various things you are encouraged to search for when searching for a trance inducer to assist you with a specific issue:

Where was the preparation for them?

Have they passed an autonomous audit?

Do you have scholastic validity in your preparation?

Is there a continuous preparing framework or a CPD framework?

Is there a supervisory framework?

Do they have protection for expert remuneration?

Do they pursue a composed morals code?

Is there a formal grumbling strategy for them?

Are they individuals from an expert body broadly perceived?

Can you call an inquiry or grievance to that body?

All BSCH individuals are prepared in great quality. We set exclusive requirements for experts of hypnotherapy. Inside the online database, you will discover various sorts of participation as laid out underneath all can, in any event, a decent degree of expertise.

Associate Member-qualified trance specialist with a go from a perceived preparing school at the Diploma/ PG Cert level.

Full Member – qualified trance specialist with a go off in any event Diploma/ PG Cert level from a perceived school of preparing and extra authorize master preparing, (for example, a Practitioner or Cognitive Behavioral level pass). Diplomate - as a full part, however, on an important clinical subject with an acknowledged paper.

Fellow-Full or Diplomatic part moved up to extraordinary administration or accomplishment from inside the general public.

To guarantee you get a confirmed and quality subliminal specialist, the different accompanying tips will manage you all the while:

Get a referral for yourself. Ask somebody you trust, similar to a companion or relative, if they have been to a trance inducer or on the off chance that they know somebody they have.

Ask for a referral from a comparative organization. A certified subliminal specialist might be prescribed by your PCP, chiropractor, analyst, dental specialist, or another restorative expert. They will likewise work with some information of your medicinal history that can enable them to prescribe a specific trance specialist in your condition.

Search online for a subliminal specialist. The Register of General Hypnotherapy and the American Clinical Hypnosis Society are phenomenal areas to start an inquiry. Visit roughly about six sites. A private site of trance inducers can offer you a smart thought of what they resemble, regardless of whether they explicitly spend significant time in anything and give some understanding into their systems and foundation. Check to see whether earlier patients have tributes. Ensure the site records the certifications of the trance inducers. Check the protection with you. On the off chance that you have psychological well-being protection, you can call them quickly and request spellbinding rehearsing specialists or another restorative workforce in your system. You can likewise get to this information on the site of your insurance agencies. Call your state mental affiliation or state guiding affiliation and solicitation the names of confirmed clinicians or approved master advisors who rundown entrancing as one of their strengths.

If required, think about a long-separation arrangement. Quality over solace is consistently the best approach with regards to your wellbeing. On the off chance that in your quick district, you experience issues finding a gifted trance inducer, extend your inquiry span to incorporate other neighboring urban communities or neighborhoods.

Ask for accreditation. No confirmed projects are gaining practical experience in hypnotherapy at noteworthy colleges. Rather, numerous trance specialists have degrees in different regions, for example, drug, dentistry, or advising, and have experienced additional hypnotherapy preparing.

Check for training in different fields, for example, medication, brain research, or social work.

Be cautious about the so-called hypnotherapy specialists. They may have gotten their doctorate from an unaccredited college on the off chance that they don't have a degree in another restorative segment.

A believable and proficient trance specialist will have proficient office offices, inside and out entrancing information, and evidence of the accomplishment of past clients.

Check whether the specialist is part of an association. The American Society of Clinical Hypnosis (ASCH) or the American Council of Hypnotist

Examiners (ACHE) are two associations expecting members to satisfy high preparing prerequisites and have sufficient aptitudes for instruction.

Looks at reviews for hypnotherapists on the internet. Sites, for example, Yelp, the Better Business Bureau, or healthgrades.com will have star appraisals and give patient audits that can help you show signs of improvement idea of how the advisor is and what the degree of fulfillment of her customers is.

Match the specialization of a the therapist with your prerequisites. Hypnotherapy can be a viable pressure and tension treatment. It can likewise profit interminable agony sufferers, hot flashes, and successive migraines. Most advisors will list their strengths on their sites. However, you ought to likewise inquire as to whether they have any experience managing your particular side effects. On the off chance that you have interminable back agony, for example, endeavor to discover a trance specialist who is likewise a chiropractor or general expert.

Ask numerous inquiries. You offer the specialist a chance to find out about you as such. You will likewise have a sentiment of how well the subliminal specialist can tune in to your prerequisites.

How long have they been prepared?

How long have they drilled?

The specialist ought to have the option to explain the differentiation between things, for example, formal and casual stupor and what awareness levels are.

Say the discoveries you are searching for to the specialist. A unique treatment plan ought to be imparted to you by the trance specialist dependent on your manifestations. Be apparent about what you plan to achieve. "I need to shed pounds" or "I need to kill ceaseless joint torment." You ought to likewise be posed inquiries about your medicinal history or any past hypnotherapy experience.

Review that you are meeting the subliminal specialist when you go to the interview to check whether they are the right fit for you.

Make sure that the trance specialist invites you.

Was the workplace spotless and amicable with the staff?

To ensure you locate the correct fit, go on a couple of discussions.

Finding a trance inducer trust your premonitions. At that point,feel free to arrange the event that you feel energetic or feel extraordinary about proceeding. Ensure you know and feel great with their methodology. Get some information about rates or costs and what number of visits your concern typically requires.

Consider pricing around. Now and then, insurance covers hypnotherapy. However, it contrasts. Check your arrangement to ensure you make an arrangement. If it is secured by your insurance, copayments can extend from $ 30 to $ 50 per visit. A subliminal specialist arrangement could cost $ 50 to $ 275 without insurance.

Hypnotic weight loss apps

1. Learning Self Hypnosis by Patrick Browning

This is a superb application to unwind following a protracted day at employment! I appreciate simply utilizing it for 30 minutes to take a portion of my day by day weight. It's exceptionally enlightening about what's mesmerizing and history. Of note is that all that you need to do in the application costs additional money.

2. Digipill

Digipill enables you to tackle your rest issue and unwind! It is additionally a precise instrument for helping you to get in shape, gain certainty, and significantly more!

3. Health and Fitness with Hypnosis, Meditation, and Music.

With this basic, however amazing application, you can get fit rapidly and keep sound. It is a helpful device that enables individuals to shed pounds by utilizing trance.

4. Harmony

Amicability is a simple method to think and unwind! You can decrease tension with this free instrument, acquire certainty, and significantly more! Free Hypnosis. This free application gives you a customized mesmerizing session of your own! It is a basic; however amazing asset for simple unwinding that contains valuable strategies and activities!

5. Stress Relief Hypnosis:

Anxiety, Relax and Sleep. You can unwind effectively with this spellbinding application! For those battling with sleep deprivation and nervousness, this free instrument is flawless.

Hypnotizing videos

Getting more fit through mesmerizing has taken off tremendously, and there are presently copious hypnotherapy sites and applications that can make a staggering decision. These spellbinding sessions are additionally a' one size fits all,' which infers that they are not customized to individual conditions, and this can make it difficult to find one that is by and by fit.

Another issue I had was the ability to hear much of the time; the voices that were once unwinding ended up irritating, which implied I was tuning in to them less and less until I halted.

I wound up edgy and disappointed, and I would not generally like to return to abstain from food, however the desire for finding something that could work for me immediately blurred.

That is the point at which I unearthed a YouTube video for David McGraw's 30-Day Challenge Ultimate Weight Loss Hypnosis. It was a 30-minute entrancing session that utilized the specialist of binaural beats and twofold enlistment. I didn't have even an inkling what that implied, yet I was entranced, and I realized I needed to attempt after tuning in to the initial ten minutes.

My concern of not having the option to tune in all the time was tackled with David McGraw since his voice covers just as being relieving, so a fraction of the time I can't generally determine what he's expression, that implies my thoughts can head off to someplace else as opposed to concentrating on the mesmerizing. NB: With entrancing, it doesn't make a difference on the off chance that you nod off as the announcements are focused at the subliminal so the cognizant can either consider different things or rest, which is extraordinary when you have a bustling life and can discover time just toward the day's end.

If you decide to give up the 30-day challenge, I suggest downloading the free MP4 version from his website, merely because YouTube will play another video afterward automatically, so if you listen at night like I do and fall asleep, you might suddenly be woken up by anything that comes up next!

As the challenge says, I decided to try it for 30 days, it's not like it cost me anything, so what can I lose? (Apart from the obvious) So this is my tale, as I said previously, I understand it's not a magic cure and I'm going to have to put some effort into it, but if it works, it's going to be so valuable to lift the heavy diet weight and continuous calorie counting.

Hypnotherapy for weight loss

If you want to lose weight, you can rely on countless diets and exercise, but in recent years you can also rely on more innovative things. Let's take a look at a step-by-step guide that explains how to use hypnosis to lose weight.

Hypnosis therapy for weight loss can be used in a way that helps control hunger and nervous cravings, especially those caused by stress and the fact that you are eating at the same time. It is time to notice how this works, how many sessions should be done, and that it is not effective.

Gastric Band Hypnosis for Rapid Weight Loss

Steps to lose weight using hypnosis

Hypnosis for weight loss is an effective treatment to reduce urges and desires and leave food vices, but the first thing to know is that it is `` help " and it can It is not a replacement.

However, studies have shown that some people have lost more than twice their weight because of hypnosis compared to those who did without treatment. Not only that, they improved their eating habits and improved their body image. On the other hand, a meta-analysis conducted by British researchers found that hypnosis can help regulate the release of peptides that control hunger and satiety mechanisms.

Therefore, hypnosis is usually aimed at nervous, emotional people, as well as those who eat at night. Very often, we eat due to lack of willpower and compensation (maybe we feel lonely, stressed and depressed, food seems to give us temporary relief). The goal of hypnosis is to break this wrong link.

This treatment does not use a pendulum that swings in front of the nose to close the eyes. The patient and the hypnotherapist will have a conversation (about 25 minutes) during the hypnosis about what the patient's goal is, what is the trigger for hunger, and what diet will be followed.

Also, experts suggest ways to deal with crisis moments when patients rely on food. Personalized therapist advice because there are different stories for each individual.

However, rather than teaching that hypnosis has no desire, you need to know that to control your desires, you understand that everything you want is not good or healthy.

Once the therapy has started, most hypnotists offer about 12 meetings. However, you have to be careful, because if after 3 or 4 sessions you have not achieved anything, this is probably not the right way. Hypnosis is not always effective and does not work for everyone equally.

Step By Step Guide To Hypnotherapy For Weight Loss

Believe. A significant part of the intensity of spellbinding lies in your conviction that you have a method for assuming responsibility for your desires. If you don't figure entrancing will enable you to change your emotions, it's probably going to have little impact.

Become agreeable. Go to a spot where you may not be stressed. This can resemble your bed, a couch, or an agreeable, easy chair anyplace. Ensure you bolster your head and neck. Wear loose garments and ensure the temperature is set at an agreeable level. It might be simpler to unwind if you play some delicate music while mesmerizing yourself, particularly something instrumental.

Focus on an item. Discover something to take a gander at and focus on in the room, ideally something somewhat above you. Utilize your concentration for clearing your leader of all contemplations on this item. Make this article the main thing that you know about.

Breathing is crucial. When you close your eyes, inhale profoundly. Reveal to yourself the greatness of your eyelids and let them fall delicately. Inhale profoundly with an ordinary mood as your eyes close. Concentrate on your breathing, enabling it to assume control over your whole personality, much the same as the item you've been taking a gander at previously. Feel progressively loose with each extra breath. Envision that your muscles disperse all the pressure and stress. Permit this inclination from your face, your chest, your arms, lastly, your legs to descend your body. When you're completely loose, your psyche ought to be clear, and you will be a piece of self-mesmerizing.

Display a pendulum. Customarily, the development of a pendulum moving to and from has been utilized to energize the center is spellbinding. Picture this pendulum in your psyche, moving to and from. Concentrate on it as you unwind to help clear your brain.

Start by focusing from 10 to 1 in your mind. You advise yourself as you check down that you are steadily getting further into entrancing. State, "10, I'm alleviating. 9, I get increasingly loose. 8. I can feel my body spreading unwinding. 7, Nothing yet unwinding I can feel.... 1, I'm resting profoundly. Keep in mind that you will be in a condition of spellbinding when you accomplish 1 all through.

Waking up from self-hypnosis. Once during spellbinding, you have accomplished what you need, you should wake up. From 1 to 10, check back.

State in your mind: "1, I wake up. 2, I'll feel like I woke up from a significant rest when I tally down. 3, I feel wakeful more.... 10, I'm wakeful, I'm new. Develop a plan. Reinventing your mind with spellbinding requires consistent redundancy. You ought to endeavor in a condition of spellbinding to go through around twenty minutes per day. While beneath, shift back and forth between portions of the underneath referenced methodologies. Attempt to assault your poor eating rehearses from any edge.

Learn to refrain from emotional overeating. One of the main things you should endeavor to do under mesmerizing is to influence yourself. You are not intrigued by the frightful nibble of food you experience issues kicking. Pick something that you will, in general, revel in like frozen yogurt. State "Dessert tastes poor and makes me feel debilitated." Repeat twenty minutes until you're prepared to wake up from the trance. Keep in mind; great eating regimen doesn't suggest you have to quit eating, simply eat less awful sustenance. Simply influence yourself to devour less sustenance, you know, is undesirable.

Write your very own positive mantra. Self-spellbinding ought to likewise be utilized to reinforce your longing to eat better. Compose a mantra to rehash in a trance state. It harms me and my body when I overeat.

Imagine the best thing for you. Picture what you might want to be more beneficial to support your longing to live better. From when you were slenderer, take a picture of yourself or do your most extreme to figure what you'd resemble in the wake of shedding pounds. Concentrate on this image under mesmerizing. Envision the trust you'd feel on the off chance that you'd be more advantageous. This will cause you to comprehend that when you wake up. Eat each supper with protein. Protein is especially valuable at topping you off and can improve your digestion since it advances muscle improvement. Fish, lean meat, eggs, yogurt, nuts, and beans are great wellsprings of protein. A steak each dinner might be counterproductive, yet in case you're eager, eating on nuts could go far to helping you accomplish your objectives.

Eat a few, modest meals daily. If you don't eat for quite a while, your digestion will go down, and you will stop fat consuming. If you expend something modest once every three or four hours, your digestion will go up, and when you plunk down for dinner, you will be less ravenous.

Eat organically grown foods. You will be loaded up with foods grown from the ground and furnish you with supplements without putting any pounds on. To start shedding pounds, nibble on bananas rather than treats to quicken weight reduction.

Cut down on unhealthy fats. It tends to be helpful for you to have unsaturated fats, similar to those in olive oil. Nonetheless, you should endeavor to limit your saturated fat and trans-fat intake. Both of these are significant factors that add to coronary illness.

Learn more about healthy cooking. In preparing meals, trans fats are common, particularly in ready to eat meals, sweets and fast food.

Saturated fats may not be as bad as trans fats. However, they might be undesirable. Major saturated fat sources include spreads, cheddar cheese, grease, red meat, and milk. The journey to weight loss is not an easy one. A person needs a lot of help and motivation to succeed. With the help of hypnotherapy, one can easily stay the course and watch the pounds melt away. Following the guide above and with a credible hypnotherapist or mastering self-hypnosis will help you in achieving your goals.

CONCLUSION

While hypnosis can provide an advantage over other weight loss methods, it is a fast fix. Research does indicate that using it with other remedies, daily exercise, and a diet might help. The study is required to evaluate the utilization of hypnosis for more weight reduction. For support, think about asking your physician for a referral to a nutritionist or other practitioner who might help you produce a weight loss plan to attain your objectives. Eating involves eating Considerable Amounts of food at a Brief period. Individuals feel as if they can't control the kind of volume of food they have. BED is a huge number of individuals around the globe. It's likely to conquer its Treatment lifestyle changes and program. While others do it, some individuals may eat sometimes regularly. Binge eating may lead therefore it's very important to address it. Binge eating that is identifying activates, planning meals that are balanced and snacks, and practicing mindful eating are approaches to decrease binge eating behaviors.

Exercise, exercise, anxiety reduction, and hydration are significant. In instances where adverse emotions or non-self-esteem activate it is essential to deal with these problems. A therapist or a physician may help. Anyone who desires support or further information, particularly should they suspect they have binge eating disorder, should talk to a health care provider. Should you suspect your child has an issue with binge eating, call your physician for referrals and guidance to mental health professionals who have experience. Reassure your child that you are there to assist or simply to listen. An eating disorder can be tricky to acknowledge, along with your child might not be prepared to admit with an issue. You are also able to encourage healthy eating habits by not using food as a reward and by mimicking your favorable relationship with exercise and food. With the support of friends, you're Loved Ones, and inviting your little one, Professionals learn how to manage stress in more healthy ways and can begin eating healthful quantities of food. Studies have found that hypnotherapy may be a powerful tool paired with even a weight management program or therapy.

To maintain your weight in check, alter your diet Complete, unprocessed foods and boost your quantity of exercise. Whether you choose to pursue not or hypnosis, which makes these lifestyle changes may result in long-term weight reduction. Lots of people struggle with overeating. There are Eating habits to improve and overcome eating disorders. Healthcare professionals such as physician's psychologists or dietitians may offer advice and counseling that will assist you to get back on the right track. Overeating can be a tough habit to break, but you may do it. Use these suggestions as a starting point to help launch a fresh routine, and be certain that you find expert assistance should you requires it. For Those Who Have concerns about your Midsection, this article should not be used by you as an excuse. While they can't be fully controlled by you your body functions, you can discover to control your eating habits and change the way you live. It's in your ability unless there's a medical condition getting on your way. It requires a lifestyle change and work, despite the odds stacked against them but people do succeed. You need to convince yourself that you're capable of before beginning any program losing weight. It is as straightforward as that. We spoke about the Vast Majority of individuals gain weight and being certain that you've noticed it is inner and psychological. It stands to reason that for change to happen, the Subconscious mind must be dealt with. The simple fact is that food culture and eating habits have to be changed to have the ability to undo this issue. The idea that it is due to too little willpower is precise what food manufacturers would like you to think that they can continue their advertising.

All the best!

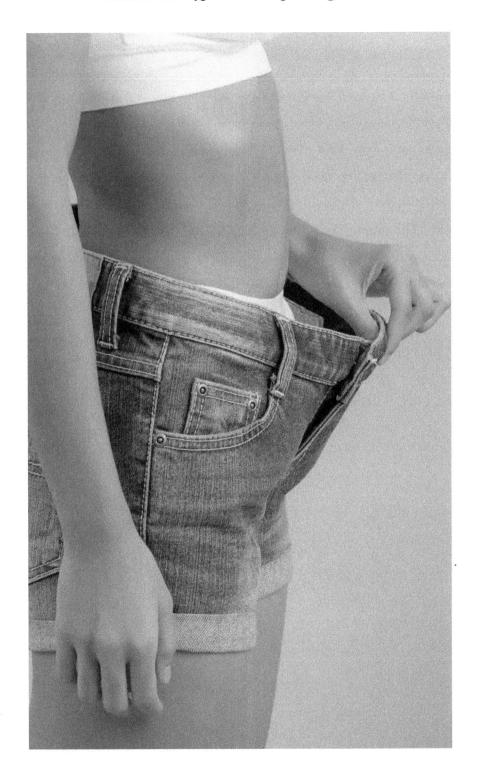

Extreme-Rapid Weight Loss Hypnosis

Eat Healthy with Rapid Weight Loss Hypnosis and Stop Food Addiction with, Meditation, Self Esteem, Powerful Habits, Mindful Eating and Self-Hypnosis.

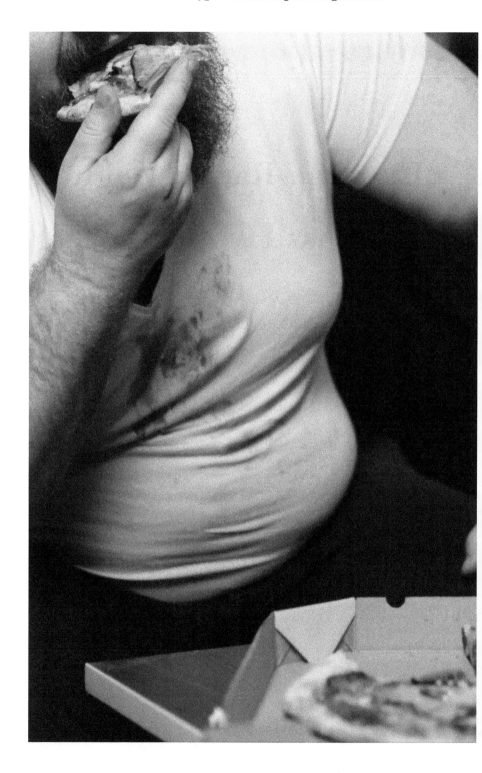

Table of Contents

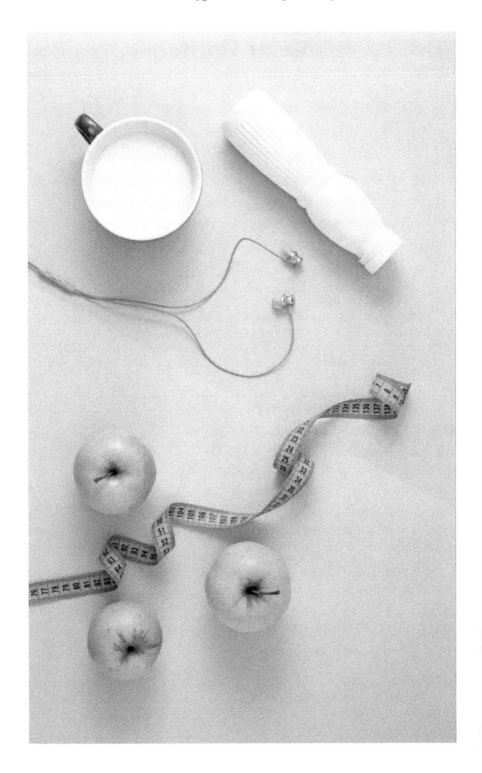

INTRODUCTION

Throughout this book, we have provided you with four different mindset exercises in order to help you lose weight. These are hypnosis, meditations, and affirmations that will make it easier for you to rewire your brain so that you're focused on achieving your goals and getting the things that you want from this life.

Make sure that you do not do any of these meditations while you're driving or operating a motor vehicle. The best place possible for these meditations is in your home, in a place where you are completely relaxed and at ease. After you know how you react to these meditations, you might be able to do them in public, such as riding a train or an airplane for long periods of travel. However, ensure that you understand how you might react, especially to hypnosis. Make sure that, as you're reading or listening to these meditations, you are focused on your breath, and keep an open mind.

What is guided hypnosis

Hypnosis has always been surrounded by misconceptions and myths. In spite of being used clinically and all the research that has been done, some continue to be scared by the assumption that hypnosis is mystical.

There are still people who think that hypnosis is a type of power held by the occult even today. The people that believe hypnosis can control minds or perform miracles are sharing the views that have been around for hundreds of years. The history that has been recorded is rich with glimpses of practices and ancient rituals that look like modern hypnosis. The Hindu Vedas have healing passes. An Ancient Egypt has their magical texts. These practices were used for religious ceremonies like communicating with spirits and gods. We need to remember that what people view as the occult was science at its finest in that time frame. It was doing exactly the same thing as modern science was doing now trying to cure human ailments by increasing our knowledge.

Finding the history of hypnosis is like searching for something that is right in our view. We can begin to see it for what it actually is – a phenomenon that is a complicated part of human existence. Hypnosis's future is to completely realize our natural hypnotic abilities and the potential we all hold inside us.

How this book can help you

It does not matter how you feel or what you're suspecting in your body, so long as you see signs that you are losing control of your body weight, then you should be evidence of your physical appearance. Seeing these signs is one thing; understanding what they mean is another thing. This book does not involve practices that you should rush or practices that you should do without a routine and a goal if you mean to change your body weight drastically. Now when it comes to knowing if your body's weight is perfect and if you have full control, then you should make sure that you have used various measures to influence your subconscious mind involved in the practices that will help to keep it in check.

To that end, you will find this book educative, and you will find valuable information meant to keep you as alert as possible in ensuring that you understand how to use this hypnotic gastric band to help to keep your body within the ideal weight and appearance. You will also learn some crucial insights that are related to hypnosis and meditation, and how you can incorporate overeating, powerful affirmations, and visualization aids to achieve your ideal weight and help to improve your relationship with food.

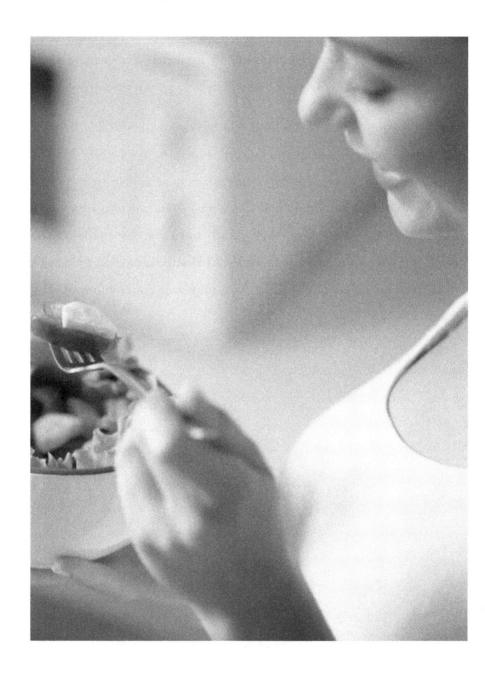

Chapter 1: Positive affirmations to enhance weight loss

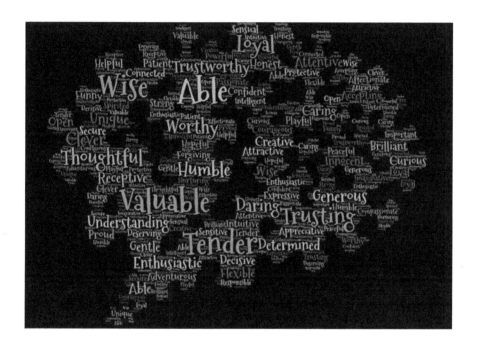

What are affirmations

Affirmations are necessary when you want to focus on another thought pattern. During affirmations, you phrase your statements positively, attach personal meaning to them, and repeat them to yourself multiple times throughout the day. Corresponding emotion helps the subconscious to understand the statements and believe them as the new status quo. At first, getting your conscious mind on board with affirmations that may seem far-fetched can be difficult. As time goes on, however, the power of these affirmations has taken root into your subconscious, and you start to believe them to be true even with your rational mind.

You should change your lifestyle if you want to have experience permanent weight loss or control. Powerful affirmations are important in helping to change your lifestyle slowly.

Thus, you should practice regular affirmations for weight loss to be able to realize your dream of losing weight. Notably, weight control is a direct function of your lifestyle because you are solely responsible for your own behavior. In other words, your weight is determined by your mental attitude, rest and sleep, physical exertion, your manner, and frequency of eating.

You can use effective weight loss affirmations to be able to initiate these measures from your mind. Thus, you should change your thinking; otherwise, no form of dieting will ever help. Weight loss affirmations are significant in your mind, as they help you to become a comfort in your desired weight.

You should also consider the words of your affirmations to ensure that you focus on the solution and not the problem. For instance, you shouldn't say "I am not that fat" because that is the problem that you're saying. Instead, you should focus on the solution and say words such as "I am getting slimmer" or "I am losing weight every day."

Try to write down some healthy weight affirmations or take a cue from the samples in this book. Repeating these words over and over, which will help to show that you are determined to take the bold step of living and fitter life.

So here are the words:

I weigh _____ pounds: this affirmation states the desired weight in your mind instantly, and as you repeat the words, you are reminding yourself about your destiny and all measures that you should take.

I will achieve my ideal weight so that I can enhance my physical fitness: you are embracing a lighter weight and improving your physical activity.

I love eating healthy food because they help me to be able to attain my ideal weight: This statement promotes healthy eating and cravings for healthy food.

I ease digestion by chewing all my food to reach my ideal weight: This affirmation is perfect to say before every meal because it guides the rate and amount of food that you consume.

I am controlling my weight by combining healthy eating, and it helps me to be able to control my appetite and my portion sizes: It is great to repeat this particular affirmation with others in front of a mirror to keep reminding your subconscious mind about your goals. Also, these affirmations work best when you're meditating or in a trance state. The combination will help to do wonders in your weight loss endeavor.

In the event that you accept the expression you are what you think, at that point life genuinely comes from your contemplations. However, we cannot depend simply on musings; we should make an interpretation of contemplations into words and in the long run into activities so as to show our expectations. This implies we must be extremely cautious with our words, expressing just those, which work towards our advantage and develop our most elevated great. Certifications help clean our musings and rebuild the dynamic of our minds, so we really start to think nothing is inconceivable. The word confirmation originates from the Latin affirm are, initially signifying "to make enduring, reinforce."

Insistences do without a doubt reinforce us by helping us put stock in the capability of an activity we want to show. When we verbally certify our fantasies and aspirations, we are immediately enabled with a profound feeling of consolation that our pie in the sky words will progress toward becoming reality. Certifications are demonstrated techniques for personal development as a result of their capacity to rework our cerebrums. Much like exercise, they raise the degree of feel-great hormones and drive our minds to frame new bunches of "positive idea" neurons. In the grouping of idea discourse activity, attestations assume a basic job by breaking examples of negative considerations, negative discourse, and, thus, negative activities.

The specialty of the verbally expressed word is basic in creating our prospects. As an educator of otherworldliness, it is my firm conviction that we impact the universe word by word. On the off chance that we manage to it our desires, it will react. When we express a sound, we radiate a sound wave into the universe. This sound wave punctures through the air and turns into a genuine item. It accordingly exists in our reality, impalpable and undetectable. No words are vacant words, as each syllable we talk connects with vitality towards or against us. On the off chance that you always state "I can't," the vitality of your words will repulse the general power against you. In any case, in the event that you state, "I can!" the universe will enrich you with the capacities to do only that. So talk away; give up your feelings of dread and cleanse your indignation, anticipate your very own future and satisfy your potential with the assertions that will transform you.

The power of repetition

Experts estimate that an average adult experiences sixty thousand thoughts in a day. Fifty thousand of these are negative. A whopping eighty percent of our thoughts are negative and unproductive. Repetitive negative thoughts can cause illness and negative outcomes in our lives. Words have a remarkable effect on our lives. They provide us with a means to share our selves and our life experiences with others. The words we regularly use affect the experiences we have in our lives. By switching up your vocabulary, you can switch up your life.

Repetition is a powerful learning tool as it is known as the "mother" of all learning. Hypnotherapists utilize repetition wisely to pack on all aspects of hypnosis. That is the same reason that relaxes the mind during repetitive hypnosis. It is said that if something frequently happens to a desired degree or amount, you will be persuaded. That is why adverts will play consistently and on repeat because repetition is about creating a familiar pattern in abundance. When you experience something over and over again, the mind understands the phenomena causing the experience to become lodged in your memory. It is repeated so many times that it becomes convincing and to some extent, nagging. Like when a chewing gum song will not leave your mind, and you keep repeating it all day long. Repetitive thought has made its way into our lives through many channels. Remember the Lord's Prayer? We can recite it by heart because it was pounded in us at an early age. So were nursery rhymes like "Row your boat." Repetition is present in songs, musical notes, prayers, chants, mantras, and many other forms of literary works. We assign weight and importance to our thoughts to determine which ones stay longer in our minds. Repetition is often reacted to as a social cue from a colleague. When people witness something done repetitively, they too begin to do it. That is how social media has become the plague it is.

When emotions are linked to certain things, repetition can be used as a trigger to awaken those emotions. The hypnotic triple is a hypnosis rule of thumb in some schools that states that something is suggested three times to culminate an effect. Not merely saying the words thrice, but also including the theme and any emotion that may be associated with it. The mind enjoys repetition because it is calming, and calming is always good. Therefore, reconstructing your subconscious mind to have dominant positive beliefs, thoughts, and habits, the more favorable your outlook on life will be.

Repetition and the Subconscious Mind

Your subconscious mind is impartial, unrelenting, and faithful. It does most of the sifting through all of our thoughts and relates them with our senses then communicates with the conscious mind through emotions. The subconscious mind collects your thoughts and stimuli from your environment and works on forming reactions to it. For example, you may see a particular person, perhaps your neighbor and feel dislike; you may even form a scowl. Yet, you have never exchanged three words with your neighbor. Why do you feel like this towards him/her? The information you fed your subconscious. The illusory truth effect is a phenomenon where something arbitrary becomes true because it was repeated over and over again when no one was paying any attention to it.

However, we do not know what the unconscious mind is working on because it does its works "behind the scenes." We cannot "sense" it hard at work, nor can we stop its processes. The good news then is that you can feed your mind with certain notions and ideals to elicit the emotions you have associated with them. Do not think, however, that the subconscious mind listens to reason; remember it remains an impartial participant in your everyday life. Take an example and remember when you tried to reason with an irrational phobia- of heights or tight spaces- for example. The conscious mind knows for a fact that there is nothing to fear, but you cannot help reacting in a particular way to these fears like getting sick, for example, and feeling dizzy.

Therefore, because your subconscious mind goes in the direction you command it; if you repeatedly affirm positive thoughts such as "I am beautiful," or "I can do this," you will automatically begin to develop a different attitude towards yourself. You will develop an inner outlook of your life which will gingerly propel you toward recognizing and taking advantage of the opportunities that come knocking at your door. The conscious mind can willingly train the subconscious mind and test the outcome using your life experiences. An excellent example of this is the power of autosuggestion. Have you heard of a vision board? They are ideas or fantasies that you pin up on a board that is strategically placed near the eye line.

The more you repeatedly see the board, the more information you are giving the subconscious mind. After a while, check to see if there are any notable improvements in your life. For most people, it takes roughly three months to see some progress, depending on how powerful your autosuggestions are.

Affirmations and Belief

Beliefs are formed by repetitive thought that has been nourished over and over for an extended period. Affirmations are positively charged proclamations or pronouncements repeated severally through the day, every day. These words are often terse, straightforward, memorable, and repetitive. Affirmations are phrased in the present tense and they lead to belief. The most crucial element of any self-improvement process is to set an intention. Muhammud Ali once said that "It is the repetition of affirmations that cause belief, and when the beliefs become deep convictions, that is when things start to happen."

Let's say you intend to shed some weight. That being the sole goal, it is paramount that all your efforts are focused on achieving it. Therefore, affirmative statements should be in the lines of, "Shedding pounds is as easy as packing them on," "I am what I eat," "A healthy mind is a healthy body," "I feel beautiful on the outside as I do on the inside," and so on. Keep in mind that not all the words you utter will yield results. For affirmations to work, they have to be coupled with visualization and a feeling of conviction. Therefore, it is advisable to focus more on positive thoughts than negative thoughts and for a prolonged period.

Remember to use words that resonate with you. The affirmations need not be empty for you. They ought to have a close relation and meaning attached to them. The proper statements for the appropriate situation goes a long way in achieving success.

You can try repeating your affirmations before you go to bed. As the brain gets ready to go on "autopilot" mode, the subconscious mind becomes more active, thereby absorbing the last bits of information for the day. Repeating affirmations before you sleep not only makes you slip into dreamland in a more confident and relaxed state but also helps to convince the mind.

You might begin to wonder why, if affirmations work, they are not used to get out of "tricky" situations. For example, if you are feeling sick, would you proceed to state, "I am cured. I am well,"? Affirmations work best with an aligned state of mind. If you believe to be well, it is more likely that you will begin to notice a decline in symptoms. If you do not believe in your affirmations, you will continue to battle through the temperature and other physical discomforts. Finding the right words to use can be a stroll in the park; however, remembering to repeat these words, severally could present itself as a challenge. The other obstacle you might face is having two conflicting thoughts. One of them is the carefully considered affirmation, while the other is a counterproductive negation. Try the best you can to disprove the negative thoughts but do not feed them time nor energy. It will be quite challenging to believe affirmations too at the beginning.

However, as time goes on, it will become easier to convince yourself. Practice makes perfect.

Affirmations seem to work because:

The act of repeating positive statements anchors your thoughts and energy, driving you toward their fulfillment

Affirmations program the subconscious mind, which in turn processes your reactions to circumstances.

The more frequently you repeat the affirmations, you become more attuned with your environment. You start seeing new opportunities, and your mind opens up to new ways of fulfilling your goals

Repetition and Hypnosis

Hypnosis aims at the subconscious part of our minds to elicit lasting behavioral changes. As we have already established, repetition relaxes the mind, and when it is employed in hypnosis, the patient arrives at a state of extreme relaxation. Hypnotic suggestions can yield positive outcomes provided the intentions are set. There are two techniques used to harness the power of repetition in hypnosis.

Listen then Repeat

To bring about success during hypnosis, you must be a good listener. When someone is speaking to you, listen cautiously to both their verbal and non-verbal cues. See what both their conscious and subconscious minds are telling you. If possible, note them down.

Then say it back to them. Repeat their suggestions back to them in the language they used. When you say something in a similar tone and style, the person tends to take it as "The Gospel." Notwithstanding they feel heard and find their thoughts acceptable when they are repeated. For example, if someone says to you "I want to shed some weight to feel more like myself," you may report back to them, "You have shed some weight, and you are feeling more like yourself." Suppose you said, "You are thin and you are feeling more like yourself." That suggestion would be utterly useless because the language used was different, therefore ineffective.

Repetitive Themes

Because themes can mean different things to different people, they become a powerful suggestive tool. Let's say a specific client always talks about one particular direction in all the meetings. Losing weight and becoming more of themselves, for instance. Take the recurrent theme and run with it. The best hypnotherapists deliver the same piece of information is a variety of ways through repetition to reinforce the principle.

You can use repetitive themes to formulate smart suggestions that are more powerful. If the subject is narrow and too specific, allow your client to broaden the topic and use the information to generalize their theme.

When appropriately applied, both techniques offer simplicity and effectiveness because hypnotherapy patients have the solutions within themselves, not to mention the brain is soothed by repetition. Therefore, the power of personal suggestion is comfortable and safe.

Using Affirmations During Self-hypnosis

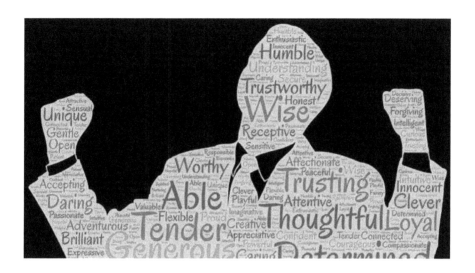

It is important to reiterate that set and setting are of paramount concern. That means that it is advisable to conduct self-hypnosis in an environment where you are not likely to be disturbed- not while operating machinery or working. Let the people in your proximity know that you will be taking a nap (because hypnosis is much like falling asleep- except with heightened sensitivity) this way; you will not be interrupted.

Step 1: Write Your Script

Ensure that the text includes the beginning that is the relaxation technique. Here, you will add the repetitive sounds and if possible, visions of the ocean, if you love the ocean waves, or the sound of falling rain, or perhaps the forest. This element will relax you, and you will begin to feel physically relaxed and comfortable.

While you are in the relaxed space, repeat your affirmations about ten to fifteen times with natural deep breaths between each mantra. Continue enjoying the comfortable space you are in, taking in the smells, sights, sounds, and temperature.

As you draw in all the senses from the space you are in, add to them the emotions triggered that particular "safe" space. As you start to feel, repeat the affirmations one more time. The conclusion of your script should include a dissociation between the trance state and the reality.

Step 2: Record Your Script

Talk slowly into the recording device. Slow your pace and remember your intention for doing this. The result will be more impactful if you slow your roll and allow the subconscious mind to absorb the words as you say them. The affirmations should include statements like, "I am 10-pounds lighter," "I have control over my body," and the like.

Step 3: Find a Quiet, Comfortable Space Where You Will Remain Uninterrupted for a Few Minutes

Keep in mind that when you are attempting a hypnotherapy session, the body temperature tends to fall below average. You can prepare for this using blankets or warm clothing. Put on your earpieces and listen to your recording.

Become aware of your eyelids getting heavier, and heavier as you gradually close your eyes. Remember to maintain a steady breathing motion- not too fast, not too slow. The breaths should be natural, do not struggle or pant for air. With every breath, feel yourself becoming more relaxed.

All the while keep your mind's eye focused on the repetitive swing of the pendulum. Count slowly downwards. Start from a comfortable number, perhaps eight or ten and with each number take a deep breath into relaxation. Believe that when you finish the countdown, you will have arrived at your ideal trance state.

Once you arrive, it is time to pay attention to your affirmations.

Step 4: Listen to the Recording Every Day

Commitment is key. As you listen to your affirmations, make sure to repeat them. It is also necessary to clear your mind before attempting to get into a hypnotic state. There are several ways of clearing the mind; for example, in the advent of hypnosis, a pendulum was used to draw the attention of the mind and maintain it. The repetitive motion of the swing causes the mind to slip into a trance state. The more you repeat the process of self-hypnosis, the easier it will become for you to reach a hypnotic state, and successfully alter your life.

The law of repetition states that repetition of behavior causes it to be more potent as each suggestion acted upon creates less opposition for the following suggestions. If you are looking to change your habits, it is of uttermost importance that you are prepared to put in the work. Reprogramming the mind towards more real life-fulfilling goals can be an uphill climb because when habits form, they become harder to break and more comfortable to follow for all organs involved.

However, all of that is learned in muscle memory. That is why repetition is emphasized. Meaning that because the mind is a muscle, it can be trained to take in more information, or rewrite existing knowledge. Just like the gym, it requires a commitment to see the results. As you practice repetition frequently, maintain actionable momentum on the subconscious and conscious levels of learning. Repetition is how successes are created.

Affirmations and your subconscious mind

Your subconscious mind has huge power in controlling your background — from the sorts of nourishment you eat to the moves you make every day, the degree of salary you gain, and even how you respond to unpleasant circumstances. All of it is guided by your intuitive convictions and elucidations.

They work best on the off chance that you adhere to a couple of basic standards: Word them emphatically, in the current state. State, "I am confident and fruitful" instead of "I will be confident and effective" in light of the fact that concentrating on a future condition does not register with your subliminal personality — it knows just this minute. Likewise, utilize positive articulations. Saying "I am not a disappointment" is registered as "I am a disappointment" since your subliminal can't process negatives.

The power of affirmations for weight loss

You should change your lifestyle if you want to have experience permanent weight loss or control. Powerful affirmations are important in helping to change your lifestyle slowly.

Thus, you should practice regular affirmations for weight loss to be able to realize your dream of losing weight. Notably, weight control is a direct function of your lifestyle because you are solely responsible for your own behavior. In other words, your weight is determined by your mental attitude, rest and sleep, physical exertion, your manner, and frequency of eating.

You can use effective weight loss affirmations to be able to initiate these measures from your mind. Thus, you should change your thinking; otherwise, no form of dieting will ever help. Weight loss affirmations are significant in your mind, as they help you to become a comfort in your desired weight.

You should also consider the words of your affirmations to ensure that you focus on the solution and not the problem. For instance, you shouldn't say "I am not that fat" because that is the problem that you're saying. Instead, you should focus on the solution and say words such as "I am getting slimmer" or "I am losing weight every day."

Try to write down some healthy weight affirmations or take a cue from the samples in this book. Repeating these words over and over, which will help to show that you are determined to take the bold step of living and fitter life.

So here are the words:

I weigh _____ pounds: this affirmation states the desired weight in your mind instantly, and as you repeat the words, you are reminding yourself about your destiny and all measures that you should take.

I will achieve my ideal weight so that I can enhance my physical fitness: you are embracing a lighter weight and improving your physical activity.

I love eating healthy food because they help me to be able to attain my ideal weight: This statement promotes healthy eating and cravings for healthy food.

I ease digestion by chewing all my food to reach my ideal weight: This affirmation is perfect to say before every meal because it guides the rate and amount of food that you consume.

I am controlling my weight by combining healthy eating, and it helps me to be able to control my appetite and my portion sizes: It is great to repeat this particular affirmation with others in front of a mirror to keep reminding your subconscious mind about your goals. Also, these affirmations work best when you're meditating or in a trance state. The combination will help to do wonders in your weight loss endeavor.

Repetition of a mantra

What are mantras and how, for what can we use them?

There are a lot of anxiety-inducing situations every day such as an important job interview, asking the boss for a pay raise, giving a lecture in front of a bunch of people, and so on. Calm breathing often turns out to be insufficient, especially in a stressful emergency situation. In this case, we need to apply another approach, the method of mantra.

What are mantras - how and for what can we use them?

There are a lot of anxiety-inducing situations every day - an important job interview, asking the boss for a pay raise, giving a lecture in front of a bunch of people, and so on. Calm breathing often turns out to be insufficient, especially in a stressful emergency situation. In this case, we need to apply another approach: the method of mantra.

10 essentials you need to know about mantras

1. The hidden possibilities of mantras

The strength of mantras honed by ancient Indian sages over many decades is concentrated, even in their ability to influence the physical level. "Mantras are like different doors that lead to the same end: each mantra is unique and thus leads to the same wisdom: to recognize that everything is one. That is, every mantra has the potential to unleash the veil of illusion and dispel the darkness. " (Deva Premal)

2. The language of mantras and their meanings

The language of mantras is Sanskrit, which is no longer considered a living language on the planet, but it is called the 'mother tongue'. We all relate to this in the same way as our language is a cellular language, a code that we understand at a very deep level. It vibrates in us something that no other language or sound can. It is a universal, cellular voice that unites us, no matter our belief system, our nationality, and our religion. You can find translated mantras, but the sounds themselves are sufficient to bring about the beneficial effects. Mantras contain deep, concentrated wisdom, meaning much more than the sum of individual words. It is therefore almost impossible to translate them accurately without losing some deeper meaning. Therefore, let us consider the translation as a guide and let the mantras work on their own.

3. The power of intention

As something is necessarily lost in the true meaning of translation, the power of our intention is very important. It is good to have a strong intention and a strong focus inside, but in fact, the effect that the mantra exerts on us is the most important. This is the true meaning of the mantra to every person who uses it. For each mantra, you will find a phrase called "Inner Focus", which broadly covers the intent of that mantra, but of course, you can also formulate an individual intent.

4. Keep the mantra with you all day

There are countless ways to make mantras part of our lives. I often carry a mantra with me all day. I would like to encourage you to do so! Carry the mantra with you throughout the day, and whenever you think of it, come back to it, the mantra being the last thing you think of before going to sleep. This is how you can truly commit to a mantra and the specific focus or theme that the mantra represents.

5. It's not necessary to chant the mantras aloud

Mantras do not necessarily have to be heard out loud. Understanding this can be a real breakthrough because it means you could carry the mantra on your own without actually chanting. So if there is a situation where you feel you need to sing the mantra out loud, concentrate on pushing it inward, carry it with you, and hold it in your being, your mind, your heart - this is the root of mantra practice when we connect with the Spirit.

6. Chant your mantras 108 times

108 is considered a very favorable number in the Vedas. According to the scriptures, we have 72,000 lines of energy in our body (the nadis), of

which there are 108 main channels of energy or major nadi that meet in the sacred heart. When a mantra is chanted 108 times, all energy channels are filled with vibrations of sound.

7. In what position should we mantra?

I recommend a comfortable position for most mantras, one with a straight back; we can relax and yet remain alert. A position that allows us presence. Because of this, a lying position is not ideal, it is harder to sing and we risk falling asleep while doing it.

8. Contemplation

Before each mantra, let's reflect on the topic of that mantra: what does it mean in our lives, do we need it, can we develop in that area, etc.? What can we sacrifice to make this quality more fully manifest in our lives? Thinking through these steps helps to refine our focus further and deepen our practice.

9. The most important "element" of the mantra is silence

Be aware that the most important "element" of the mantra that we reach through the mantra is the silence. This is seemingly a paradoxical thing: the silence after singing is what our soul dives into and is reborn. This silence represents the transcendent, the eternal, the reality, and understanding or achieving this is the ultimate goal of mantra practice.

10. Importance of repetition and practice

The essence of mantra practice is not to get over it quickly and then return to our usual daily routine. The point is to practice and to integrate the mantras into our lives. Wherever we go, whatever we do, the mantras accompany us. This is the benefit of true mantra practice. It helps and supports the path of our lives. The power of mantras is multiplied by repetition and devotional practice. The more pleasure we can bring into our practice, the more pleasure we get. Like real friends, mantras can help you through times of need and stress.

How do we use mantras in everyday life?

The method is simple! We need to talk to ourselves - of course, what we say matters. I may surprise you by saying that it's enough to repeat only three words in every situation when you feel under pressure. These three words are: "I am excited."

Yes, I know, it is not what you have expected from me. You may wonder why you should use a statement that is not so 'positive'. Harvard University published a study in the Journal of Experimental Psychology, in which scientists claim that striving to overcome anxiety may not be the best solution in such situations. Instead of trying to calm ourselves down, it can be more useful to transform stress into a powerful and positive emotion, such as excitement. Because positive feelings produce quite similar physical symptoms as anxiety, hence, we wouldn't have great difficulties switching the stress to excitement. Enthusiasm is a positive emotion, besides, it is easier to cope with. The study also recalls earlier research that mild anxiety can even be a motivator for specific tasks. So it is worth using the energy generated by stress to increase our efficiency, instead of trying our best to suppress it. To turn fear-based anxiety into a positive feeling, repeat for 60 seconds to yourself, "I am excited." This mantra "redraws" the picture of a stressful situation into something we happen to be waiting for - which is far less exhausting than trying to calm ourselves down.

Using different mantras is very important to me, and I use them daily for my meditations or just for relaxation. You can also use them whenever you are sad, or you don't know where you belong to what you have to do with your life. They help you to see through and view yourself. If you have been to a place where people have been singing or chanting, you will know how much power and energy there is in a particular word.

One of the best-known mantras is "Aum" or "Oum." It is found among Hindus but also in Buddhism. Followers believe this mantra purifies the soul and helps to release negative emotions. This mantra is also known as a sign of the "quick eye" chakra.

If you want to reach the best result, sing AUM loudly so that its sound vibrates in your ears and soaks your entire body. It will convince your outer sense, give you greater joy and a sense of success. When singing AUM loudly, "M" should sound at least three times as long as "AU". When repeating "AUM", imagine that life energy, divine energy flows through you through the crown chakra. The breath that flows through your nose is very limited. But if you can imagine that there is a large opening at the top of your head, and life energy, cosmic energy is flowing into your body through that opening, you will undoubtedly be able to accelerate the purification of your nature, strengthen your aspiration and hunger for God, Truth, Light, and Salvation.

There are many ways to sing "AUM". If we repeat "AUM" with the immense power of the soul, then we enter into the cosmic vibration where creation is in perfect harmony. If the soul completely repeats the "AUM", we become one with the Cosmic Dance; we become one with God the Creator, God the Maintainer, and God the Transformer (Saunders, n. d.).

Repeat the following mantras to obtain a change in your life:

- I want to experience being part of the universe.

- I wish my slim shape was restored.

- I desire and undertake the necessary changes to restore my slim shape.

(Include 300 affirmations)

⇨ I am healthy, wealthy and clever

⇨ I let go of the illness, i am not ill

⇨ Thanks to my creator and everyone in my life.

⇨ I am grateful for all the bounty that I already enjoy

⇨ Every day I grow energetically and vibrantly

⇨ I only give my body the necessary nutritious food

⇨ My body is my temple

⇨ You can always maintain a healthy weight

⇨ I deserve to enjoy perfect health

⇨ Act to be healthy

⇨ I respect my body and am willing to exercise

⇨ Affirmation For Rapid And Natural Weight Loss

⇨ My body is beautiful and healthy

⇨ I choose healthy and nutritious foods

⇨ I like to exercise and I do it frequently

⇨ Losing weight is easy and even fun

⇨ I have confidence in myself

⇨ I am now sure of myself

⇨ I feel confident to succeed

⇨ From day to day, I am more and more confident

⇨ I am sure to reach my goal

⇨ I want to be a noble example

⇨ I believe in my value

⇨ I have the strength to realize my dreams

⇨ I am really adorable

⇨ I trust my inner wisdom

⇨ Everything I do satisfies me deeply

⇨ I trust the process of life

⇨ I can free the past and forgive

⇨ No thought of the past limits me

⇨ I get ready to change and grow

⇨ I am safe in the Universe and life loves me and supports me

⇨ With joy I observe how life supports me abundantly and provides me with more goods than I can imagine.

⇨ Freedom is my divine right

⇨ I accept myself and create peace in my mind and my heart

⇨ I am a loved person and I am safe.

⇨ Divine Intelligence continually guides me in achieving my goals

⇨ I feel happy to live

⇨ I create peace in my mind, and my body reflects it with perfect health

⇨ All my experiences are opportunities to learn and grow

⇨ I flow with life easily and effortlessly

⇨ My ability to create the good in my life is unlimited

⇨ I deserve to be loved because I exist

⇨ I am a being worthy of love

⇨ I dare to try and I'm proud of it

⇨ I choose to really love myself

⇨ I love myself and accept myself completely

⇨ I am ready to try new things

⇨ There are things I can already do, I just need to start even though I'm not ready yet

⇨ I am much more capable than I think

⇨ As I love myself, I allow others to love me too ...

⇨ I accumulate more and more confidence in myself

⇨ I am unique and perfect as I am

⇨ I am wonderful

⇨ I'm proud of everything I've accomplished

⇨ I do not have to be perfect, I just need to be myself

⇨ I feel able to succeed

⇨ I give myself permission to go out of my role as a victim and take more responsibility for my life

⇨ The past is over, I now have control of my life and I move

⇨ I am my best friend

⇨ I am able to say "no" without fear of displeasing

⇨ I choose to clean myself of my fears and my doubts

⇨ Fear is a simple emotion that can not stop me from succeeding

⇨ Every step forward I make increases my strength

⇨ My hesitations give way to victory

⇨ I want to do it, I can do it

⇨ I am capable of great things

⇨ There is no one more important than me

⇨ I may be wrong but that I can handle it

⇨ With confidence, I can accomplish everything

⇨ I allow myself to have a lot of fun

⇨ I deserve to be seen, heard and shine

⇨ I deserve love and respect

⇨ I choose to believe in myself

⇨ I allow myself to feel good about myself and trust myself

⇨ I reduce measures quickly and easily

⇨ I can maintain my ideal weight without many problems

⇨ My body feels light and in perfect health

⇨ I'm motivated to lose weight and stay

⇨ Every day I reduce measures and lose weight

⇨ I fulfill my weight loss goals

Gastric Band Hypnosis for Rapid Weight Loss

⇨ I lose weight every day, and I recover my perfect figure

⇨ I eat like a thin person

⇨ I treat my body with love and give it healthy food

⇨ I choose to feel good inside and out

⇨ I feed myself only until I am satisfied, I don't saturate my food body

⇨ I know how to choose my food in a balanced way.

⇨ I feed slowly and enjoy every bite.

⇨ I am the only one who can choose how I eat and how I want to see myself.

⇨ It is easy for me to control the amounts of what I eat.

⇨ I learn to have habits that lead me to my ideal weight.

⇨ Being at my ideal weight makes me feel healthy and young.

⇨ My body is very grateful and quickly reflects all the care I have with him.

⇨ My body reflects my perfect health.

⇨ I feel better every day

⇨ Being at my ideal weight motivates me to do other things that I like.

⇨ The human body is moldable, and I am the (the) artist of my body.

⇨ Every day I eat with awareness.

⇨ I consume the calories needed to have an ideal weight and a healthy body.

⇨ Every day I like the way I feel.

⇨ My slender body makes me feel, agile, light (and) and strong at the same time.

⇨ I know how to properly calculate the portions my body needs to feel satisfied.

⇨ I can achieve everything that I propose.

⇨ No one can do this for me, only I can make the best version of me, inside and out.

⇨ I am the inspiration for other people.

⇨ I like how the clothes look on my slender body.

⇨ I am strong physically and mentally.

⇨ No one can get me out of my motivation for being a healthy and slender person.

⇨ Being at my ideal weight fills me with energy.

⇨ My metabolism is faster every day thanks to the food I eat.

⇨ I love my new lifestyle.

⇨ I am getting better and better.

⇨ I accept all the blessings of the universe.

⇨ Reality is created from my thoughts.

⇨ I decide to choose thoughts that will have a positive impact on my life.

⇨ The biggest job to do is on my own.

⇨ I am open to all new experiences of life.

⇨ I am free to think what I want.

⇨ I will achieve great things.

⇨ I will be the best to accomplish this task.

⇨ I value myself because I am a good person.

⇨ I have full possession of my means.

⇨ I hide all the negative things that I can not change.

⇨ I love myself a lot because I am a good person.

⇨ I am able to climb mountains.

⇨ I am able to reverse any reality.

⇨ I totally approve of everything I do.

⇨ All my decisions are taken in hindsight and these are good for me.

⇨ I am unique.

⇨ I believe in myself inconsiderately.

⇨ I think positively.

⇨ Understanding is one of my biggest qualities.

⇨ I have all the qualities in me to reach my ends.

⇨ I am determined to deal with all situations.

⇨ I am a man capable of exceeding my limits.

⇨ I am a totally unique person with great qualities.

⇨ I am a good person and I deserve happiness.

⇨ All my decisions are good at different levels.

⇨ Serenity is an integral part of me.

⇨ I am the person I think I am.

⇨ I agree with the people around me and trust my colleagues.

⇨ Self-esteem is my main quality.

⇨ My life is plenty of confidence .

⇨ I am a confident person who keeps getting better every day.

⇨ I trust my choices and I move in that direction.

⇨ I erase in my life all the people who prevent me from achieving happiness.

⇨ I control my choices and my life.

⇨ I am responsible for my positive mental state.

⇨ I deserve a fulfilling life.

⇨ What I feel is healthy.

⇨ Trust in me is my first quality.

⇨ I attract good in my life.

⇨ I will offer everything I have given.

⇨ Love is present, it is enough that I believe in it.

⇨ I am aware that my friends love me.

⇨ I have a family and relatives who surround me.

⇨ I have a fulfilling social life.

⇨ I am love.

⇨ I make the world better every day.

⇨ I like family time.

⇨ I take the time necessary to show my entourage how important they are to me.

I love them.

⇨ I am able to take time for myself and for my loved ones.

⇨ Compassion is part of me.

⇨ I am able to give forgiveness.

⇨ I practice benevolence with conviction to help my entourage to evolve.

⇨ I am able to question myself and understand.

⇨ I choose to do what I like.

⇨ I believe in love.

⇨ I let my heart speak.

⇨ I am able to let people love me.

⇨ I like others and others love me in return.

⇨ I accept that others can love me.

⇨ Fusional / passional love is coming into my life.

⇨ The people I love love me back.

⇨ I am able to give love to others.

⇨ If I give others love, they make it exponentially.

⇨ I am able to attract the person I want.

⇨ My sentimental relationships are strong and fulfilling.

⇨ I'm ready to fall in love.

⇨ I give a lot because I love this person

⇨ Love is in me.

⇨ Love is only an extension of my fulfillment.

⇨ Joy filled me and filled my life.

⇨ The people around me are filled with love and I benefit from it.

⇨ I'm falling in love.

⇨ The waves around me tell me that love is present.

⇨ Hidden love is a real love.

⇨ I love to love a person.

⇨ I take the front and reveal my love.

⇨ Like a magician I chose to give love all around me.

⇨ I like people even my enemies.

⇨ I receive love as I pass it.

⇨ My life is happy and joyful.

⇨ I feel good with this person.

⇨ My relationship is passionate and I feel fulfilled.

⇨ I give everything to my companion to make her as happy as possible.

⇨ Love is an integral part of my life.

⇨ Passion paces my choices.

⇨ I am able to let my heart make decisions.

⇨ My heart is full of happiness.

⇨ Harmony is present in me.

⇨ I love life and life loves me.

⇨ I understand my feelings and accept them.

⇨ I deserve to find love

⇨ I am endearing and open to others.

⇨ I am able to open myself to others.

⇨ I am able to confess the things that I feel.

⇨ I only feel positive things with people around me.

⇨ I only transmit positive to those around me.

⇨ I focus on the things that make me happy.

⇨ I believe in the power of attraction.

⇨ I concentrate my efforts on what I really want.

⇨ Money is a reward.

⇨ I am able to get as much money as I want.

⇨ Money is a form of remuneration that takes different forms and I am already rich.

⇨ I think so I create.

⇨ What I am doing now will be beneficial in the future.

⇨ My efforts will pay very soon.

⇨ I attract all that looks like me like a magnet.

⇨ I am very prosperous.

⇨ I live well financially.

⇨ Money is abundant in my life.

⇨ Everything I do brings me closer to freedom and prosperity.

⇨ I really believe in the strength of attraction.

⇨ My money is proportional to my happiness.

⇨ The money I earn is a symbol of my beliefs.

⇨ I believe in my ability to become rich quickly.

⇨ My productivity, my knowledge and my knowledge allow me to attract money easily.

⇨ I will earn money very quickly.

Repr I reprogram my mind so that it attracts abundance .

⇨ Every day that rises, my wealth increases.

⇨ I am in full in abundance.

⇨ I agree to take risks to generate my fortune.

⇨ I am a successful billionaire.

⇨ I have the ability to generate large amounts of money.

⇨ I accept and focus on actions that bring me closer to wealth.

⇨ Financial freedom is an integral part of my personality.

⇨ I accomplish my goals and bring me closer to success and abundance every passing day.

⇨ Abundance allows me to be fulfilled and enjoy life.

⇨ The wealth I create is not necessarily just paper money.

⇨ My professional and personal success will give me abundance and financial freedom.

Positive Affirmations of The Morning

⇨ The world is created to offer us beautiful things.

⇨ I become what I imagine.

⇨ I create my future.

⇨ I am ready to have a very good day.

⇨ I am the captain of my spirit and the master of my soul.

⇨ I will have a very good day.

⇨ I literally believe in the power of positive thinking.

⇨ I respect people because they are like me.

⇨ I am in good shape.

⇨ Every day offers a new range of possibilities.

⇨ My mind is only a reflection of what I think.

⇨ I am a happy person and ready to move on.

⇨ All I wish is going back into my life without my noticing it.

⇨ The experiences of life are magical, every day I learn new things.

⇨ Today will be a day full of twists and turns.

⇨ I know exactly what I'm going to do with my day.

⇨ I am literally happy during this day.

⇨ I am determined to perform this morning routine.

⇨ Joy is already present in my life, it is enough for me to open my eyes to see it.

⇨ Every waking morning, I leave the bed with enthusiasm and happiness in relation to my life and my day to come.

⇨ I am fulfilled and feel very good about myself.

⇨ My dreams are my reality.

⇨ Energy is abundant in me.

⇨ I smile at every opportunity.

⇨ Smiles are the first thing I do when I wake up.

⇨ The morning is the best time of the day.

⇨ I have confidence in the future.

⇨ I exceed my limits every day a little more.

⇨ Sport is part of me.

⇨ I am able to create the body I want.

[YOUTUBE VIDEO] Positive affirmations of the morning

Positive affirmations »Work«

⇨ I know how to push myself to get what I want.

⇨ My job is the hidden part of my success.

⇨ I like the moments spent at work.

⇨ I am doing today the tasks entrusted to me without putting off to the next day.

⇨ I'm acting now to create the future I want now.

⇨ I work a lot on my projects with an inconsiderate joy.

⇨ My work is a moment of pleasure where I learn to surpass myself.

⇨ I am able to let go for better results.

⇨ I give myself breaks.

⇨ The rewards are already there, I just can not see them for the moment.

⇨ I assume all my responsibilities with kindness.

⇨ I stay positive even in the face of the most negative things.

⇨ My work is done with rigor.

⇨ Conviction dictates my work.

⇨ My motivation is the key to my success.

⇨ My work is governed by my determination.

⇨ My work is the key to my success.

⇨ I am master of the direction of my life.

⇨ My job allows me to get what I want most.

⇨ Productivity is abundant in my actions.

⇨ I am aware of my ability to work.

⇨ I'm doing a good job.

⇨ I demonstrate to my boss my abilities.

⇨ My actions are proof of my determination at work.

⇨ Difficulty is an element of motivation to show who I really am.

⇨ My work is organized and I am my action plan.

⇨ Concentration is a quality that I have that allows me to do my job well.

⇨ I am able to make decisions at work.

⇨ My personal success is present.

⇨ My professional life is rich and fulfilling.

⇨ Every moment spent at work brings me closer to my goals.

⇨ My life is a success.

⇨ I have clear ideas about my future.

Claims To Lose Weight Quickly And Naturally

⇨ You can maintain an ideal weight.

⇨ Help your body recover and maintain your ideal weight.

⇨ I can eliminate the excess that my body has accumulated.

⇨ You can return your body to its original state.

⇨ Make your body do what it takes to maintain your ideal weight.

⇨ My body is clever.

⇨ My body maintains an ideal weight without much effort.

⇨ My body knows what to use.

⇨ My body knows what to remove.

⇨ My body knows what it needs and how to get it.

⇨ My body can maintain its ideal weight, without me intervening.

⇨ My body tells me that I should eat and when.

⇨ My body knows what foods I should consume.

⇨ Food is just food and has no power over me.

⇨ I allow my body to take advantage of all the good things about food.

⇨ I allow my body to eliminate what it does not need.

⇨ I allow my body to stop accumulating.

⇨ I know that I am always well fed.

⇨ My body is healthy by nature.

⇨ I allow my body to recover its natural health.

⇨ I allow my body to maintain its natural state of health.

⇨ My body stays healthy naturally.

⇨ MY body knows how to maintain your health and your ideal weight.

⇨ My body knows what it takes to stay healthy.

⇨ I can maintain my ideal weight.

⇨ I can maintain my ideal weight easily and effortlessly.

⇨ I can eliminate excesses from my body easily.

⇨ I can keep my body healthy and in perfect condition.

⇨ I can maintain my weight naturally.

⇨ I can easily maintain my ideal weight.

⇨ My body is healthy and perfect.

⇨ Nothing outside of me can affect the health and natural state of my body.

⇨ Nothing outside of me has control over my weight and my figure.

⇨ Nothing outside of me can affect my weight.

⇨ Nothing outside of me can affect my health.

⇨ Nothing outside of me can influence my weight and my health.

⇨ Every day my body is healthier.

⇨ Every day my body is healthier and beautiful.

⇨ Every day my body regains its natural beauty.

⇨ Every day my body is more beautiful and healthy.

Gastric Band Hypnosis for Rapid Weight Loss

⇨ Every day my body is more beautiful.

⇨ Every day in every way my body is healthier and beautiful.

⇨ Every day my body eliminates what it doesn't need.

⇨ Every day my body stays healthier.

⇨ Every day my weight stays at its ideal level.

⇨ Every day my body retains its ideal weight.

⇨ Every day my body is healthier.

⇨ Right now I am losing weight.

⇨ Right now I am removing excess fat.

⇨ Right now my body is eliminating the bad.

⇨ Right now my body is eliminating the negative.

⇨ Right now my body is regaining its ideal weight

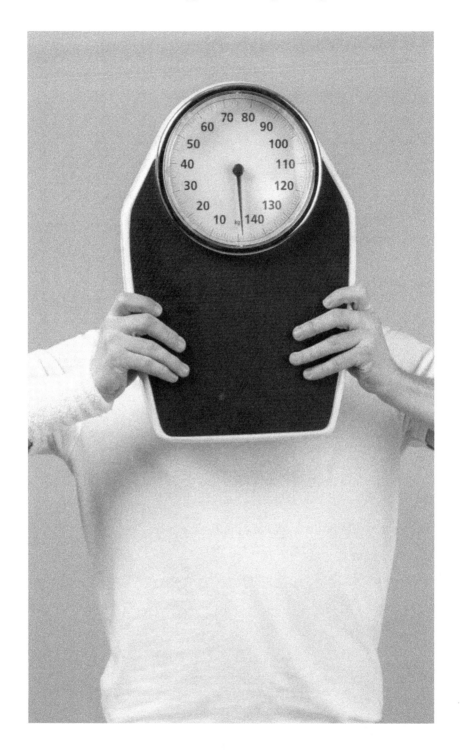

Chapter 2: Deep sleep meditation

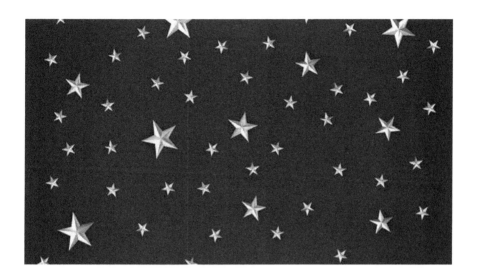

Deep-sleep meditation and weight loss

Y ou are laying in a completely comfortable position right now. Your body is well rested, and you are prepared to drift deeply into sleep. The deeper you sleep, the healthier you feel when you wake up.

Your eyes are closed, and the only thing that you are responsible for now is falling asleep. There isn't anything you should be worried about other than becoming well-rested. You are going to be able to do this through this guided meditation into another world.

It will be the transition between your waking life and a place where you are going to fall into a deep and heavy sleep. You are becoming more and more relaxed, ready to fall into a trance-like state where you can drift into a healthy sleep.

Start by counting down slowly. Use your breathing in fives in order to help you become more and more asleep.

Breathe in for ten, nine, eight, seven, six, and out for five, four, three, two, and one. Repeat this once more. Breathe in for ten, nine, eight, seven, six, and out for five, four, three, two, and one.

You are now more and more relaxed, more and more prepared for a night of deep and heavy sleep. You are drifting away, faster and faster, deeper and deeper, closer and closer to a heavy sleep. You see nothing as you let your mind wander.

You are not fantasizing about anything. You are not worried about what has happened today, or even farther back in your past. You are not afraid of what might be there going forward. You are not fearful of anything in the future that is causing you panic.

You are highly aware within this moment that everything will be OK. Nothing matters but your breathing and your relaxation. Everything in front of you is peaceful. You are filled with serenity and you exude calmness. You only think about what is happening in the present moment where you are becoming more and more at peace.

Your mind is blank. You see nothing but black. You are fading faster and faster, deeper and deeper, further and further. You are getting close to being completely relaxed, but right now, you are OK with sitting here peacefully.

You aren't rushing to sleep because you need to wind down before bed. You don't want to go to bed with anxious thoughts and have nightmares all night about the things that you are fearing. The only thing that you are concerning yourself with at this moment is getting nice and relaxed before it's time to start to sleep.

You see nothing in front of you other than a small white light. That light becomes a bit bigger and bigger. As it grows, you start to see that you are inside a vehicle. You are laying on your bed, everything around you is still there. Only, when you look up, you see that there is a large open window, with several computers and wheels out in front of you.

You realize that you are in a spaceship floating peacefully through the sky. It is on auto-pilot, and there is nothing that you have to worry about as you are floating up in this spaceship. You look out above you and see that the night sky is more gorgeous than you ever could have imagined.

All that surrounds you is nothing but beauty. There are bright stars twinkling against a black backdrop. You can make out some of the planets. They are all different than you would ever have imagined. Some are bright purple, others are blue. There are detailed swirls and stripes that you didn't know were there.

You relax and feel yourself floating up in this space. When you are here, everything seems so small. You still have problems back home on Earth, but they are so distant that they are almost not real. There are issues that make you feel as though the world is ending, but you see now that the entire universe is still doing fine, no matter what might be happening in your life. You are not concerned with any issues right now.

You are soaking up all that is around you. You are so far separated from Earth, and it's crazy to think about just how much space is out there for you to explore. You are relaxed, looking around. There are shooting stars all in the distance. There are floating rocks passing by your ship. You are floating around, feeling dreamier and dreamier.

You are passing over Earth again, getting close to going back home. You are going to be sent right back into your room, falling more heavily with each breath you take back into sleep. You are getting closer and closer to drifting away.

You pass over the earth and look down to see all of the beauty that exists. The green and blue swirl together, white clouds above that make such an interesting pattern. Everything below looks like a painting. It does not look real.

You get closer and closer, floating so delicately in your small space ship. The ride is not bumpy. It is not bothering you.

You are floating over the city now. You see random lights flicker on. It doesn't look like a map anymore like when you are so high above.

You are looking down and seeing that gentle lights still flash here and there, but for the most part, the city is winding down. Everyone is drifting faster and faster to sleep. You are getting closer and closer to your home.

You see that everything is peaceful below you. The sun will rise again, and tomorrow will start. For now, the only thing that you can do is prepare and rest for what might be to come.

You are more and more relaxed now, drifting further and further into sleep.

You are still focused on your breathing, it is becoming slower and slower. You are close to drifting away to sleep now.

When we reach one, you will drift off deep into sleep.

How to practice deep-sleep meditation for weight loss

Sleep is incredibly important, but sometimes falling asleep can be difficult if we are not in the right mindset.

For this activity, we are going to take you through a visualization that will help ensure that you can get a deep sleep. It's important before falling asleep to relax your mind so that you can travel gently throughout your brain.

Start off by noticing your breath. Breathe in through your nose and out through your mouth. This is going to help calm you down so that you are able to breathe easier.

Begin by breathing in for five and out for five as we count down from twenty. Once we reach one, your mind will be completely clear. Each time a thought passes in, you will think of nothing. You will have nothing in your sight, and you will only think with your mind.

Make sure that you are in a comfortable place where you can sink into the space around you. Let your body become heavy as it falls into the bed. Keep your eyes closed and see nothing in front of you but darkness.

Each time a thought comes in, keep pushing it away. Breathe in through your nose and out through your mouth.

Remember to breathe in for five and out for five. Keep an empty mind and be ready to travel through a journey that will take you to a restful place.

You see nothing in front of you, it is completely dark and you feel your body lifting gently up like a feather. You are light against the bed, and nothing is keeping you down. Continue to feel your body rise higher and higher. You are floating in space. There's black nothingness around you. You are gently drifting around.

You can see a few stars dotting the sky so far away, but for the most part, you see nothing. You feel yourself slowly moving through space.

Your body is light and free, and nothing is keeping you strapped down. You're not afraid in this moment.

You are simply feeling easy and free. Breathe in and out, in and out.

You start to drift more towards a few planets, throughout your journey in space. You can really see now that you are up in the highest parts of the galaxy. You see out of the corner of your eye that you can actually catch a glimpse of Earth. You start gently floating towards it, having to put no effort in at all as your body is like a space rock floating through the stars.

Nothing is holding you down.

Nothing is violently pushing you either. Everything that you feel is a gentle and free emotion. You get closer and closer to Earth now and can see all the clouds that surround you. You start to move down, and you gently enter into the cloud area.

Normally gravity would pull you down so fast, but right now you're just simply a gentle body drifting through the air. You get closer and closer to the land. You can see some birds here and there and a few cars and lights on the ground beneath you.

You pass all of this. Gently floating over a sleepy town.

Look down and let your mind explore what is it that you see down there. What is it that is in front of your eyes? What do you notice about this world around you as you continue to go closer and closer to home?

You are gently drifting throughout the sky. You can see trees beneath you. Now, if you reached your hand down, you'd even be able to gently feel a few leaves on the tops of the tallest trees. You don't do this now because you're just concerned with continuing to float through the sky. That's all that you really care about in this moment.

You're getting closer and closer and closer to home now, almost ready to fall asleep.

You start to see that there is a lake.

You gently float down to the surface of the lake, and you land right in a boat. Your body is a little bit heavier now. You feel it relax into the bottom of the boat. Nothing around you is concerning you right now. You feel no stress or tension in any part of your body. You are simply floating through this space now. The boat starts to gently drift on the lake. It is dark out now and you look up and see all the stars in the sky. All of this reminds you of the place that you were just a few moments ago. You start to drift closer and closer to sleep.

Do you feel as the tension leaves your body? You are peaceful throughout. You are not holding on to anything that causes you stress or anxiety. You are at ease in this moment. Everything feels good and you have no fear. You drift around in the water now for a little bit longer. You can see everything so clearly in this night sky. Just because it is dark does not mean that it's hard to see. The moon casts a beautiful glow over everything around you. You can feel the moon charging your skin. As you drift closer and closer to sleep, you feel almost nothing in your body now. You continue to focus on your breathing. You are safe, and you are at peace.

You are calm, and you are relaxed. You feel incredible in this moment.

The boat starts to lift from the water. You feel as it gets higher above the water. You are even heavier now. Now you are completely glued to this comfortable surface as the boat starts to fly through the sky. You can look down and see that the city beneath you has drifted to sleep. You're getting closer and closer to home now. You can actually see your home beneath you. The boat gently takes you to your front door, and you float right in. No need to walk or climb stairs. You simply float in and straight to your bed.

You fall delicately into your bed with your head resting nicely on a pillow.

Here you are, in this moment, so peaceful and so relaxed. You are completely at ease. There's nothing that stresses you out or causes any anxiety or tension now. You are simply a body that is trying to fall asleep.

As we count down from 20, you will drift off to sleep. You will be in a very relaxed state where nothing stresses you out. You're not concerned with things that happened in the past, and you aren't going to stay up in fear of what might happen tomorrow, you are asleep. You are relaxed.

Breathe in and out. Breathe in and out.

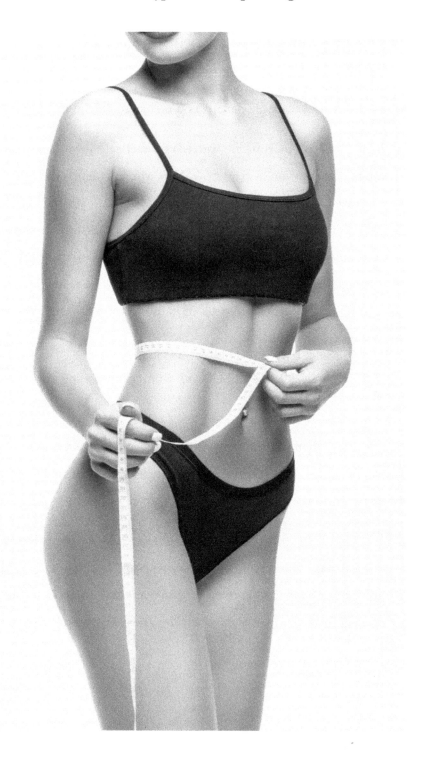

Chapter 3: Hypnotic gastric band

What is a gastric band

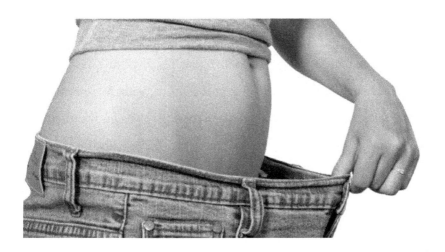

A gastric band is a silicone device commonly used to treat obesity. The device is normally placed around the upper part of your stomach to help decrease the food that you're eating. On the upper part of the stomach, the band makes a relatively smaller pouch. It fills up quickly and slows your consumption rate. The band shows you whenever you make healthy food options, reduce appetite, and limit food intake and volume.

However, it leaves you with a difficult option of bariatric surgery, which is a drastic step that carries risks and pains like any other gastrointestinal surgical operation. You should not experience these challenges when you can take a simple and less invasive approach to achieve the same results as in a surgical gastric band.

How to create a gastric band using hypnosis

If you would like to lose some weight without using surgery, then the hypnotic gastric band is the best tool for you. The hypnotic gastric band is the natural healthy eating tool that will help to control your appetite and your portion sizes. In this sense, hypnosis plays a significant role in helping you to lose weight without having to go through the risk that comes with surgery.

It is a subconscious suggestion that you already have, a gastric band comes intending to influence the body to respond by creating a feeling of satiety. It is now available in a public domain that dieting does not help to solve lifestyle challenges that are needed for weight loss and management.

Temporary diet plans are not effective while maintaining continuous plans are difficult. Notably, these plans are going to totally deprive you of your favorite foods, since they're too restrictive. Deep down within you, you might have a problem with your body's weight since diets have not worked for you in the past.

If you want to try something that will be able to provide a positive edge for you, then you should be able to control your cravings around food hypnotically. By reaching this point, you must try hypnosis, which has proven some results in aiding weight loss.

Benefits of hypnosis vs surgery

If you would like to lose weight without starvation or yo-yo dieting, then hypnotic gastric band is the ultimate resort for you. This gastric band does not require surgery but only meditation and hypnosis. Therefore, it offers numerous benefits that make it the solution to rapid weight loss and craving healthy food.

It is pain-free: As opposed to the physical gastric band, the hypnotic gastric band does not require surgery which is associated with pain and routine follow-ups. Therefore, you do not need to worry about the risks you need to take as no physical operation will be done on your body. You only need to hypnotize and utilize the hypnosis to work on your body weight.

100% safe: As hypnosis is a non-invasive, non-surgical, and safe technique so is the hypnotic gastric band whose mechanism is initiated in your subconscious mind. Through the practice, there are no expected dangers and you learn about self-awareness and the course of your life.

Time-efficient: You do not need to wait for your vacation to acquire a hypnotic gastric band. The tool does not affect your schedule as hypnosis can be combined with most of your day to day activities. You do not need time off to adjust the band or report complications

No meal replacement or dieting: With hypnotic gastric band, you do not need to stop eating your most enjoyable food. Instead, you develop a principle that makes you feel in control and enable you to lose weight consistently and naturally without dieting. You just exercise and unlock the power in you to make positive changes in life.

No complications: The fact that no surgery is performed in hypnotic gastric surgery puts away the worry about future complications. The ease in your mind plays a significant role in focusing your mind on the things that matter such as visualization and meditation. This way, you are able to put off negative thinking and live your life fearlessly and positively.

Helps discover your hidden potential: The use of hypnosis and meditation makes you learn about how to utilize the power of your mind in changing your perception and erasing negative thoughts. Similarly, you become capable of helping not only with weight loss but also with other psychological and social aspects such as confidence. In this case, hypnosis helps plant a subconscious suggestion in your mind making it stick and become a strong idea.

Cost-Effective: Hypnotic gastric band does not snatch away your working time making you fully productive at your workplace with no deductions. In the same way, there are no costs in hypnosis and meditation as opposed to the physical gastric band. Positively living your life actually substantially adds to your savings.

Weight loss through hypnosis

Now, as I am walking down the beach, I will come to an area with unpleasant bells written by me in the sand. Those labels have been given to me in the past. Those labels are the labels that have held me back in the past from reaching my true capacity and from reaching my true power. I see those labels in the sand, and I begin to use my leg to clean them and use my legs to wash it off and clean the area with sweeping. With my feet, I erase the words away with every stroke of my feet, and I watch as the water comes to the shore to clear them away and clear all this around me.

Those words mean nothing to me; they do not exist again because I was the only one that saw them. I turn them around, and I work a little way down the beach. I feel more confident and taller. I come to the middle of a large rock sitting in the middle of the sand, and on this rock, there is a little pick. I pick it up, and I begin to write all the things that I want about my life. I begin to write all the things that I want about my weight. I am writing all the things that describe me. I am writing that I am confident, I am talented, and I am accomplished. And that I am a good person. I write as many words as possible that describe me.

I write things like positive, attractive, and capable I look at all the words that I have written on this rock and I know that I am a great person. I begin to recall all the moments whereby I felt confident. I think of the time that I felt confident, and I recall those feelings again. I visualize those convenient moments in my life, and what it felt like, what it sounded like, and I then realize what it smells like. I believe this positive moment in my life. I think of the times where I felt confident in my life.

I feel those feelings. I picture those moments again, and I make the colors brighter and more vivid. I feel those feelings of confidence and pride, and I turn off the sounds and the smells. I get back into those moments where I was feeling so confident and powerful that I was feeling so confident in myself and all the things that I was doing. I am confident in the way I look. I am confident in the way I dress, and I'm confident in the way I act. I am confident in my relationship. I am confident in the relationship that I have with the members of the opposite sex. I am confident in the relationship that I have with my family with my friends and my coworkers.

Things come to me easily, with the way I talk to people. Conversations come out fluently from my mouth, and people respect what I have to say. I am strong and respected, and everyone around me sees me as confident and capable I take a look at myself, and I see that I am full of positive energy. I am the one that is radiating how everyone sees me. Everyone around me sees the positive energy in me, not only the people around me, but I also respect myself. I stand tall and strong. I stand proud of myself. I know that I can accomplish whatever I put my mind to accomplish. All I am seeing are positive things in my life.

I have practical and creative ideas, and I fill my mind with positive energy. I drop the future and go forward with confidence. I imagine myself one year from now, and I imagine the person that I will grow up to be. When I imagine this image, I will not be able to recognize the person that I once was. I have accomplished great things in the past year, great things that will help me to reach my capabilities.

My confidence has enabled others to look at me with great confidence and respect. I enjoy talking with people, and they're interested in what I have to say. My career is going great, and I can voice my ideas and opinions to other people because they value them. The relationship with my friends and families are great. Most of my friends and families come to seek advice from me because they hold me in high esteem. I look at myself, and I see how positive I am. I can point others in the right direction that they should go. I have faith in myself. I have great ideas, and I know that my family and friends respect my ideas, and they know my values too. I hold my head high and I know that nothing can bring me down. I stand tall and strong because I know that I am an accomplished, beautiful, capable and confident person.

Different techniques hypnosis, meditation, affirmations: 3 steps placing, tightening, removal

Placing

In this meditation, you will learn how to walk along a beautiful beach walk, allowing you and deeply relax.

Follow me on this mental vacation as we place an emotional and mental and gastric band around your stomach, which will allow you to feel a full as soon as you eat exactly as much food as you need.

So, get into a comfortable seated position, on your favorite spot, so that you are undisturbed for the rest of this session. As you relax, the gastric band will become more powerful and influential over your life. Take a big deep breath, relax, and then exhale the tension and worry as you close your eyes. Feel your body already slowing down. Take another breath and let to go with a sigh of relief. This moment is for you to practice your new lifestyle, of being full, at the perfect time. Now say to you with faith, "overeating is impossible for me."

Now breathe into the truth of these words as you breathe them out into reality. You are creating a smaller stomach. Relax and breathe and then use the power of your imagination to visualize a beautiful beach with white sand, reflecting in the sunlight. It looks like snow. You can see the turquoise waters fading to a deep blue as the ocean goes deeper.

Look down into the sand where you stand, and notice the beautiful bits of shells with all different colors and textures as you see dried seaweed scattered about something that catches your eye buried into the sand, it is your preferred color. So as you get closer, you will see that it is a small yet thick band that is as big around as your fist, and it just so happens that it is the most vivid version of your favorite color. The brightness of this hue brings you joy. The curious, round band, flashing of your most beloved color choice is called the gastric band

It is placed around the top of your stomach, cinching down the amount your stomach can hold. So, it makes your stomach feel smaller, which gives you that feeling of fullness that you've had enough to eat. This band only exists in the medical world. But, you can get the same results, using the power of your mind, by placing the band within and around your stomach in this relaxing session.

But before you do this, try to walk along a beach (this beach is gorgeous), carrying around your gastric band. Feel and notice the band in your hand and notice the texture, the width, and the weight of the band.

Feel your feet entering the sand and allow yourself on each step to relax more and more. Notice the powdery texture, dispersing under your feet, and allow it deeply soothe you. Feel the ocean breeze, and smell the salty air. As you walk, you will get tired. A perfect chair has appeared just for you, facing the ocean. So have a seat and recline backward with your gastric band in your hand. Familiarize yourself with its shape and size. It is like a small belt that can be tightened and loosened.

Will it work for me ?

Normally, the conscious mind is receptive to suggestions, because it normally analyzes it.

With hypnosis, you will be able to reach your desired weight, become healthier, and stay in shape for life with the right mindset. You will be able to empower your mind to accept suggestions in a deep and relaxed state. This way, you will be able to reframe your thinking patterns because of all the principles of suggestion and disassociation. With the hypnotic gastric band, you will be able to use suggestions to influence a different response from your body triggered by sensory data to be able to create a new reality. The suggestions will be to provide a guideline for you to follow without questioning or critiquing.

Ultimately, this power will be able to allow you to reframe and reshape your perception regarding a specific behavior. The complex network in your brain has many different interpretations of the world around you, and the most unhelpful and negative thoughts have worked their way into that network.

Thus, you become susceptible to uncontrolled unconscious urges, like overeating and ignoring bodyweight concerns. Hypnotic gastric band will help you to be able to dampen and overcome all those uncontrolled thoughts, believes, and suggestions that are helping you alter your behavior. Types of gastric banding techniques used in hypnotherapy

Sleeve gastrectomy - This procedure involves physically removing half of a patient's stomach to leave behind space, which is usually the size of a banana. When this part of the stomach is taken out, it cannot be reversed. This may seem like one of the most extreme types of gastric band surgeries, and due to its level of extremity, it also presents a lot of risks. When the reasons why the sleeve gastrectomy is done and gets reviewed, it may not seem worth it. However, it has become one of the most popular methods used in surgery, as a restrictive means of reducing a patient's appetite. It is particularly helpful to those who suffer from obesity. It has a high success rate with very few complications, according to medical practitioners. Those who have had the surgery have experienced losing up to 50% of their total weight, which is quite a lot for someone suffering from obesity. It is equally helpful to those who suffer from compulsive eating disorders, like binge eating. When you have the procedure done, your surgeon will make either a very large or a few small incisions in the abdomen. The physical recovery of this procedure may take up to six weeks. (WebMD, n.d.)

• Vertical banded gastroplasty - This gastric band procedure, also known as VBG, involves the same band used during the sleeve gastrectomy, which is placed around the stomach. The stomach is then stapled above the band to form a small pouch, which in some sense shrinks the stomach to produce the same effects. The procedure has been noted as a successful one to lose weight compared to many other types of weight-loss surgeries. Even though compared to the sleeve gastrectomy, it may seem like a less complicated surgery, it has a higher complication rate. That is why it is considered far less common. Until today, there are only 5% of bariatric surgeons perform this particular gastric band surgery. Nevertheless, it is known for producing results and can still be used in hypnotherapy to produce similar results without the complications.

• Mixed Surgery (Restrictive and Malabsorptive) - This type of gastric band surgery forms a crucial part of most types of weight loss surgeries. It is more commonly referred to as gastric bypass and is done first, prior to other weight-loss surgeries. It also involves stapling the stomach and creates a shape of an intestine down the line of your stomach. This is done to ensure the patient consumes less food, referred to as restrictive mixed surgery, combined with malabsorptive surgery, meaning to absorb less food in the body.

Chapter 4: Mindful eating habits

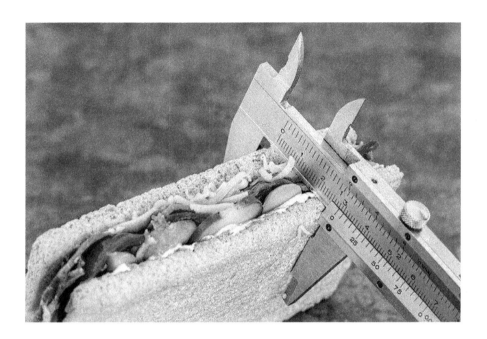

What are eating habits

Healthy Eating Habits That Everyone Needs to Have

Avoid emotional eating

Emotional eating has been a challenge for most people. Anytime time you get mad, you find that your immediate solution is to start eating. In that state, you might be prompted to overeat which is harmful to your body. You find that we go through some challenging situations and we lack appropriate measures to handle some of these struggles. Meditation can bring you in a state of calmness. In that state, you get to identify the various challenges that you are facing. It allows you to establish the cause of some of those challenges and upon identifying them, you can easily come up with a possible solution. Asides from emotional eating, you find that there are other alternatives to use to solve the problem at hand. One of the good eating habits you can utilize is avoiding emotional eating. In this case, you find other alternatives that you can engage in that can help you solve the problem. When you do this, you will realize a lot of improvement in your eating habits and attaining some of the body goals that you have will be possible.

Chewing slowly

Chewing helps an individual in weight loss. While chewing, you can take your time after taking a bite. Ensure that all the food present in your mouth has been properly chewed before swallowing. This process of slowly chewing ensures that food is properly ingested. Some of the digestion processes begins to take place in the mouth; for instance, starch is digested in the mouth, as you chew, some of this starch is digested. If you end up chewing too fast, not all the starch will be digested in the mouth, so it's carried to places where it cannot be digested. As a result, you find that the starch will not be useful to the body since it has not undergone the process of digestions. When this happens recurrently, you get to pile up a lot of unnecessary food components in your body that is not processed. Eventually, you start adding extra weight as the excess food gets converted into fats. To avoid this, you need to slowly and properly chew the food that you consume. That way, it is beneficial to your body.

Eating small portions of food

Consuming large amounts of food in a few sessions is not recommended. You find that in a day, an individual consumes the right portion of the food that they should take. However, the food may not help them at all. What one needs to do is take little portions of the required amount. In this case, you can decide to eat after every two hours. During this time, your body is able to properly utilize each amount of food consumed. If it needs to be converted into energy, almost all the consumed food is utilized. When you do this, you barely have excess food in your system, and you can easily manage that which is available. You will be surprised by how this habit can help you in losing weight. The idea is to eat well by ensuring that you consume the right portion of food at different sessions. This process ensures that no food goes to waste. It also prevents the incidences of overeating. You will find that you will hardly eat when full. Once you adopt this type of eating habit, you only eat when necessary, and the food that you consume helps your body.

Having a meal plan

It is very easy to come up with a meal plan. All you need to do is to identify the foods that you need to eat and the time you want to consume them. While coming up with a meal plan, you can consider one diet or combine different diets as long as what you consume is beneficial to your body. A plan directs you on the particular meals to consume on a given day and prevents you from eating food substances that you should not consume at a given time. You find that most times we make rush decisions into purchasing items without evaluating if they are necessary or not. The majority of the decisions that we make in life are an impulse. This happens since we have not taken some time to properly plan and prevent some of these incidences from occurring. A plan is essential in helping one avoid making some impulse decisions that they will end up regretting later on. When it comes to eating, we at times, make impulse decisions to purchase food that we do not need at a particular moment. With a good meal plan, you can avoid some of these purchases.

Drinking water

The biggest percentage of the human body is composed of water. We need water to survive and go about our various activities in life. The majority of the time we ignore this factor and barely drink water. You find that an individual can go for days without taking water, yet it is a basic need. One may argue out that water can be present in the foods that we consume, but that may not be enough for your body. At times it is good to take proper care of your body by ensuring that you stay hydrated. There are some diseases that you can prevent when you take proper care of your body. Water has also been recommended for having a glowing skin. When you are well hydrated, your body is in the right shape and responds positively. As you consume water, it allows you to get rid of the waste products that are present in your body. It also facilitates the process of digestion and in turn, allows proper functioning of the body. In the process of eliminating waste, water can help in weight loss and ensuring that you are in the right shape.

Reduce your carb intake

Carbohydrates are mainly composed of sugars. You find that when you consume them in excessive quantities, the sugar levels in your blood stream increases. It is in excess, the majority of it is converted into fats, and you end up adding extra weight. One of the best ways to lose weight is to avoid that which made you gain weight in the first place. Excessive intake of carbohydrates can also result in some diseases such as diabetes and heart complications. To avoid them, ensure that you eat just the required amount of carbohydrates.

Develop an eating routine

Do you have an eating schedule? You find that the majority eat food only when they feel hungry or when they have the time to eat. When you have a busy schedule, and you are trying to balance doing a variety of things, you may not have adequate time to eat. You find that most of the time you prefer takeout's or snacks that are unhealthy. When you keep upholding such habits, you may find it difficult to eat well. There are certain times when you should eat a certain quantity of food.

For instance, as you start your day in the morning, breakfast is the most important meal. It ensures that you are energetic to carry out the businesses of the day. Most people do not take breakfast and mainly focus on eating much at night. Eating at that time is not beneficial since the food consumed is not used by the body, and the majority of eating becomes waste. There are very few activities happening at night, and you don't require as much energy as you would during the day. It is good to come up with an eating schedule that you follow strictly.

Eat plant-based meals

Vegan meals tend to have lots of nutrients that are beneficial to our bodies. We have health practitioners encouraging individuals to turn to consume plant-based meals. Currently, lifestyle diseases have been on the rise. We rarely look at what we are consuming. Healthy eating has been a topic of discussion for a long time, and some seem to take it with much seriousness while others just ignore and face the repercussions later on. At the beginning of each year, we have people making resolutions that they will change their diet, but they barely do anything about it. Or find that you start out really well for the first few weeks, then you end up backsliding. As you walk along the street, you come across a food trunk selling junk, and all you want to do is have some. Once you decide to eat plant-based meals, you require some discipline that ensures you follow the plan to the latter. At times you will feel tempted, but you have to do all that you can so that the urge does not overpower you. With time you will get used to them, and you will find it easy to eat them regularly.

Look for some healthy snacks

Any time we hear the word snack mentioned anywhere, you immediately think of refined carbohydrates or processed foods. That is a misguided belief since we also have some healthy snacks. You could get some unsweetened yogurt, groundnuts, cashew nuts, or some roasted kales. These are some of the healthy snacks that you can consume and can be beneficial to your body. In case you are an individual who likes snacking a lot, or if you barely have time to eat actual meals within the day, you can look for some healthy snacks. If you are used to taking unprocessed foods and sugars, you can replace them with a healthy but sweet snack. For a person who loves sugars, some fruits can be a good alternative. They are both sweet and nutritious when consumed. Nuts are also nice when used as a snack; they are delicious and will add value to your body. The idea that snack can only be unrefined carbohydrates or processed foods should end since there are plenty of healthy snacks that are available. Most times we just choose to go for junk only because of the sugars they contain, and we end up ignoring some sweet but healthy snacks that contain natural sweetness.

Eat health foods at social gatherings

Different types of foods are served in functions. Social gatherings offer a good time to bond with each other and make merry. They are designed to be a fun moment where one relaxes from a busy week. In such functions, all you want to do is celebrate and utilize each moment. In the process of having fun, eating some good food might be your major agenda. You find that you consume a lot of food in one sitting, and most of what you consume is not helpful to the body. At times you find that you are eating just because every other person is eating and not because you are hungry. Your brain sends certain signals, and you find yourself filling your plate to capacity even if you are unsure whether you will finish. To avoid such incidences from occurring, ensure that you serve the portion that you need. On the other hand, try and ensure that you serve yourself more of the plant-based foods available. Avoid filling your plate with too many carbohydrates since they are not helpful when taken in excess. Ensure that you take more fruits and salads that add value to your body.

Mindful eating

You need to increase your awareness of eating if you want to lose weight by trying to make changes to your eating habits. Here are the steps to take to increase your awareness of eating.

First of all, look at the food and what you're about to eat. Focus on the food just focus on it and ask yourself, "do I really want to eat this food into my body." Then pay attention to every bite of the food eat. Eat mindfully so that it will be easier to digest. Do not overeat it. After eating, notice how your body feels and notice how the food affected your digestive system. Ask yourself, did it agree with you. Notice how you felt when eating a lump of high meat versus how it felt like when eating a raw vegetable snack versus or when eating a candy bar snack.

Principles of mindful eating

Here are a couple of tips for getting you started.

Start with one meal. It requires some investment to begin with any new propensity. It very well may be difficult to make cautious eating rehearses constantly. However, you can practice with one dinner or even a segment of a supper. Attempt to focus on appetite sign and sustenance choices before you start eating or sinking into the feelings of satiety toward the part of the arrangement— these are phenomenal approaches to begin a routine with regards to consideration.

Remove view distractions place or turn off your phone in another space. Mood killers such the TV and PC and set away whatever else —, for example, books, magazines, and papers— that can divert you from eating. Give the feast before your complete consideration.

Tune in your perspective when you start this activity, become aware of your attitude. Perceive that there is no right or off base method for eating, yet simply unmistakable degrees of eating background awareness.

Focus your consideration on eating sensations. When you understand that your brain has meandered, take it delicately back to the eating knowledge.

Draw in your senses with this activity. There are numerous approaches to explore. Attempt to investigate one nourishment thing utilizing every one of your faculties. When you put sustenance in your mouth, see the scents, surfaces, hues, and flavors. Attempt to see how the sustenance changes as you cautiously bite each nibble.

Take as much time as necessary. Eating cautiously includes backing off, enabling your stomach related hormones to tell your mind that you are finished before eating excessively. It's a fabulous method to hinder your fork between chomps. Additionally, you will be better arranged to value your supper experience, especially in case you're with friends and family.

Rehearsing mindfulness in a bustling globe can be trying now and again; however, by knowing and applying these essential core values and techniques, you can discover approaches to settle your body all the more promptly. When you figure out how much your association with nourishment can adjust to improve things, you will be charmingly astounded — and this can importantly affect your general prosperity and wellbeing.

Formal dinners, be that as it may, will, in general, assume a lower priority about occupied ways of life for generally people. Rather, supper times are an opportunity to endeavor to do each million stuff in turn. Consider having meals at your work area or accepting your Instagram fix over breakfast to control through a task.

The issue with this is you are bound to be genuinely determined in your decisions about healthy eating and eat excessively on the off chance that you don't focus on the nourishment you devour or the way you eat it.

That is the place mindfulness goes in. You can apply similar plans to a yoga practice straight on your lunch plate". Cautious eating can enable you to tune in to the body's information of what, when, why, and the amount to eat," says Lynn Rossy, Ph.D., essayist of The Mindfulness-Based Eating Solution and the Center for Mindful Eating director. "Rather than relying upon another person (or an eating routine) to reveal to you how to eat, developing a minding association with your own body can achieve tremendous learning and change."

From the ranch to the fork — can help you conquer enthusiastic eating, make better nourishment choices, and even experience your suppers in a crisp and ideally better way. To make your next dinner mindful, pursue these measures.

Practice mindful eating everyday

We eat mindlessly. The principal explanation behind our awkwardness with nourishment and eating is that we have overlooked how to be available as we eat. Careful eating is the act of developing a receptive familiarity with how the nourishment we eat influences one's body, sentiments, brain, and all that is around us. The training improves our comprehension of what to eat, how to eat, the amount to eat, and why we eat what we eat. When eating carefully, we are completely present and relish each chomp - connecting every one of our faculties to really value the nourishment. Past simple tastes, we see the appearance, sounds, scents, and surfaces of our nourishment, just as our mind's reaction to these perceptions.

The precepts of care apply to careful eating too; however, the idea of careful eating goes past the person. It likewise incorporates how what you eat influences the world. When we eat with this comprehension and understanding, appreciation and empathy will emerge inside us. Accordingly, careful eating is fundamental to guarantee nourishment supportability for who and what is to come, as we are persuaded to pick nourishments that are useful for our wellbeing, yet in addition useful for our planet.

It is outstanding that most get-healthy plans do not work in the long haul. Around 85% of individuals with heftiness who shed pounds come back to or surpass their underlying load inside a couple of years. Binge eating, passionate eating, outside seating, and eating because of nourishment longings have been connected to weight put on and weight recovers after effective weight reduction. Interminable presentation to stress may likewise assume an enormous job in gorging and heftiness. By changing the manner in which you consider nourishment, the negative sentiments that might be related to eating are supplanted with mindfulness, improved poise, and positive feelings. At the point when undesirable eating practices are tended to, your odds of long-haul weight reduction achievement are expanded.

Steps to Mindful Eating

1. Watch your shopping list

Shopping mindfully, – purchasing sound nourishments that are reasonably delivered and bundled – is a significant piece of the training. One thing you will probably find about careful eating is that entire nourishments are more dynamic and heavenly than you may have given them acknowledgment for.

2. Figure out how to Eat Slower

Eating gradually does not need to mean taking it to limits. All things considered, it is a smart thought to remind yourself, and your family, that eating is not a race. Setting aside the effort to relish and make the most of your nourishment is perhaps the most advantageous thing you can do. You are bound to see when you are full, you'll bite your nourishment more and consequently digest it all the more effectively, and you'll likely end up seeing flavors you may some way or another have missed.

3. Eat when Necessary

It might take some training, however, locate that sweet spot between being eager and being ravenous to the point that you need to breathe in a dinner. Additionally, tune in to your body and get familiar with the distinction between being physically eager and sincerely ravenous. On the off chance that you skip dinners, you might be so anxious to get anything in your stomach that your first need is filling the void as opposed to making the most of your nourishment.

4. Enjoy your Senses

The vast majority partner eating with simply taste; and many eat so carelessly that even the taste buds get quick work. Be that as it may, eating is a blessing to a greater number of faculties than simply taste. When you are cooking, serving, and eating your nourishment, be mindful of shading, surface, fragrance, and even the sounds various nourishments make as you set them up. As you bite your nourishment, take a stab at distinguishing every one of the fixings, particularly seasonings. Eat with your fingers to give your feeling of touch some good times. By drawing in various faculties, the entire experience turns out to be significantly more completely fulfilling.

5. Keep off Distractions

Our day by day lives are brimming with interruptions, and it is normal for families to eat with the TV booming or one relative or another tinkering with their iPhone.

Think about making family supper time, which should, obviously, be eaten together, a hardware-free zone. This does not mean eating alone peacefully; careful eating can be a great mutual encounter. It just means do not eat before the TV, while driving, at the PC, on your telephone, and so on. Eating before the TV is for all intents and purposes the national hobby, however, simply consider how effectively it empowers careless eating.

6. Stop when you are Full

The issue with astounding nourishment is that by its very nature, it tends to be difficult to quit eating. Eating gradually will enable you to feel full before eating excessively, but on the other hand, it is imperative to be mindful of segment size and tune in to your body for when it starts disclosing to you it has had enough. Gorging may feel great at the time; however, it is awkward a short time later and is commonly not beneficial for the body. With a little practice, you can locate the without flaw spot between eating enough, however not all that much.

Careful eating does not need to be an activity in super-human focus, but instead a straightforward promise to acknowledging, regarding and, most importantly,getting a charge out of the nourishment you eat each day. It very well may be drilled with serving of mixed greens or frozen yogurt, doughnuts or tofu, and you can present it at home or at work. While the center turns out to be the means by which you eat, not what you eat, you may discover your thoughts of what you need to eat moving significantly for the better as well.

Hypnosis to create mindful eating habits

In addition to helping you encourage yourself to eat healthier while discouraging yourself from eating unhealthy foods, you can also use hypnosis to help encourage you to make healthy lifestyle changes. This can support you with everything from exercising more frequently to picking up more active hobbies that support your wellbeing in general.

You may also use this to help you eliminate hobbies or experiences from your life that may encourage unhealthy dietary habits in the first place. For example, if you tend to binge eat when you are stressed out, you might use hypnosis to help you navigate stress more effectively so that you are less likely to binge eat when you are feeling stressed out. If you tend to eat when you are feeling emotional or bored, you can use hypnosis to help you change those behaviors, too.

Hypnosis can be used to change virtually any area of your life that motivates you to eat unhealthily or otherwise neglect self-care to the point where you are sabotaging yourself from healthy weight loss. It truly is an incredibly versatile practice that you can rely on that will help you with weight loss, as well as help you with creating a healthier lifestyle in general. With hypnosis, there are countless ways that you can improve the quality of your life, making it an incredibly helpful practice for you to rely on. In the following chapters, we are going to explore how you can use hypnosis as a way to support you with weight loss, as well as improving your wellbeing overall.

CONCLUSION

E ating involves eating Considerable Amounts of food at a Brief period. Individuals feel as if they can't control the kind of volume of food they have. BED is a huge number of individuals around the globe. It's likely to conquer its Treatment lifestyle changes and program. While others do it, some individuals may eat sometimes regularly. Binge eating may lead therefore it's very important to address it. Binge eating that is identifying activates, planning meals that are balanced and snacks, and practicing mindful eating are approaches to decrease binge eating behaviors.

Exercise, exercise, anxiety reduction, and hydration are significant. In instances where adverse emotions or non-self-esteem activate it is essential to deal with these problems. A therapist or a physician may help. Anyone who desires support or further information, particularly should they suspect they have binge eating disorder, should talk to a health care provider. Should you suspect your child has an issue with binge eating, call your physician for referrals and guidance to mental health professionals who have experience. Reassure your child that you are there to assist or simply to listen. An eating disorder can be tricky to acknowledge, along with your child might not be prepared to admit with an issue. You are also able to encourage healthy eating habits by not using food as a reward and by mimicking your favorable relationship with exercise and food. With the support of friends, you're Loved Ones, and inviting your little one, Professionals learn how to manage stress in more healthy ways and can begin eating healthful quantities of food. Studies have found that hypnotherapy may be a powerful tool paired with even a weight management program or therapy.

To maintain your weight in check, alter your diet Complete, unprocessed foods and boost your quantity of exercise. Whether you choose to pursue not or hypnosis, which makes these lifestyle changes may result in long-term weight reduction. Lots of people struggle with overeating. There are Eating habits to improve and overcome eating disorders. Healthcare professionals such as physician's psychologists or dietitians may offer advice and counseling that will assist you to get back on the right track. Overeating can be a tough habit to break, but you may do it. Use these suggestions as a starting point to help launch a fresh routine, and be certain that you find expert assistance should you requires it.

It requires a lifestyle change and work, despite the odds stacked against them but people do succeed. You need to convince yourself that you're capable of before beginning any program losing weight. It is as straightforward as that. We spoke about the Vast Majority of individuals gain weight and being certain that you've noticed it is inner and psychological. It stands to reason that for change to happen, the Subconscious mind must be dealt with.

CPSIA information can be obtained
at www.ICGtesting.com
Printed in the USA
BVHW041514190321
602997BV00010B/506

9 781801 655125